YOGA AS INTEGRATIVE MEDICINE

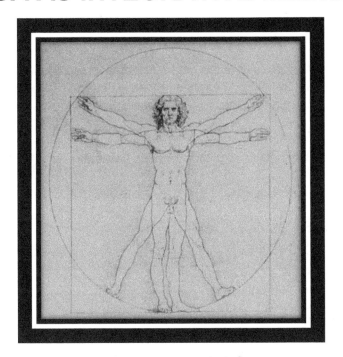

YOGA SUTRAS
MEET
GRAY'S ANATOMY

MARY DURYEA MD, C-IAYT, E-RYT 500

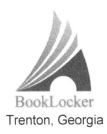

BookLocker
Trenton, Georgia

Print ISBN: 978-1-64719-866-4
Ebook ISBN: 978-1-64719-867-1

Published by BookLocker.com, Inc., Trenton, Georgia.

Printed on acid-free paper.

BookLocker.com, Inc.
2021

First Edition

Library of Congress Cataloguing in Publication Data
Duryea MD, C-IAYT, E-RYT 500, Mary
Yoga As Integrative Medicine by Mary Duryea MD, C-IAYT, E-RYT 500
Library of Congress Control Number: 2021920410

Dedicated to Mother Earth, the sapphire jewel, now in need of intensive care. Let us make sure she does not end up in hospice. Your choices, your voice, and your vote have influence. Future generations also deserve to experience the beauty and the bounty of nature.

Also dedicated to my children Karl, Kelsey, and Tessa, my grandson Leo, and any future grandchildren. My hope is this book will have a positive influence and provide a means to remember my love.

"We are not human beings having a spiritual experience.
We are spiritual beings having a human experience."

– Pierre Teilhard de Chardin

TABLE OF CONTENTS

Chapter One:
East Meets West

"We live in succession, in division, in parts, in particles. Meantime within man is the soul of the whole; the wise silence; the universal beauty, to which every part and particle is equally related; the eternal ONE."

~ The Over-Soul by Ralph Waldo Emerson

An Invitation to Contemplation

Yoga has become immensely popular in recent years and gained status around the world. Millions of people strongly embrace the practice as a form of physical fitness and stress reduction. Images of yoga now permeate our modern society, with media depictions being commonplace compared with twenty years ago. Numerous studios and teacher training programs have sprung up worldwide. Yoga has been commercialized through social media, exotic retreats, fashionable clothing, cool mats, and new props. Being widely practiced around the world, yoga has justifiably earned dual citizenship, at home both in the East and in the West. Fortunately, the newly emerging field of yoga therapy is also becoming an accepted part of Western integrative medicine.

Why are so many people embracing yoga and willing to spend time and money on it? Because adopting yoga practices as lifestyle habits may improve one's sense of well-being and contentment, as well as fill a void in self-nurturing that exists for many of us. Often, right from the start, the physical practice of yoga will initiate a greater sense of health and ease in the body. With continued time, commitment, and a deeper understanding of the teachings of yoga, a sense of mental, emotional, and spiritual well-being may also emerge. This ability for an individual to self-nurture through the practice of yoga is likely to improve overall health and quality of life.

Having been around for thousands of years in its various forms, yoga is clearly here to stay. Yoga appeals to many people with a wide variety of backgrounds. Why is this true? What are some of its traditional teachings? What are the tools used to achieve a more holistic progression toward improved health? What exactly is being taught and how does it work? What are some potential cautions related to yoga practices? These are some of the questions I address in this book through the lens of my experience as a Western medicine physician.

I want to appeal to healthcare providers who recommend yoga to learn more about it, so yoga becomes less esoteric. I also want to appeal to inquisitive yoga teachers who wish to integrate Western medical concepts into yoga teachings, and perhaps pass this knowledge on to their clients. In parts of this book, yogic concepts are correlated with teachings of anatomy and physiology from Western medicine. I have endeavored to use straightforward language so that both the Western medical terms and the yogic concepts make sense to the general reader. My goal for this book is to help medical professionals better understand yoga, to help the yoga practitioner better understand Western medicine, and to help everyone appreciate the power of yoga to enhance the human experience.

I also want to advocate for yoga therapy as a key component of integrative medicine, which combines traditional Western medicine with other techniques to improve the overall health of the individual. The National Institutes of Health (NIH) website states:

> "Integrative healthcare often brings conventional and complementary approaches together in a coordinated way. It emphasizes a holistic, patient-focused approach to healthcare and wellness—often including mental, emotional, functional, spiritual, social, and community aspects—and treating the whole person rather than, for example, one organ system. It aims for well-coordinated care between different providers and institutions."[i]

Note that this definition does not involve just physical well-being, but also "mental, emotional, functional, spiritual, social, and community aspects." Yoga addresses each of these aspects of an individual. I find it particularly gratifying that "spiritual" was included in this NIH definition. Spirituality was originally the primary focus and most important aspect of yoga. Traditionally, spirituality has not been emphasized in Western medicine. Yoga may help fill this "spirituality gap" in modern medical healthcare. And although yoga addresses this topic, yoga is not a religion and can be practiced by anyone regardless of religious beliefs.

I envision yoga therapy as a growing part of integrative medicine, in which a variety of professionals each bring their own unique skill set for care of the patient. Integrative medicine is rather like a healthcare "stew." If a variety of high-quality ingredients—that is, qualified healthcare professionals—is incorporated into healthcare, then the final product, namely the health of the patient, benefits. Yoga also empowers patients to take an active role in their own self-care. Once learned, yoga can be practiced by virtually anyone, anywhere, anytime and takes little space, time, or money.

In this informative book, I share my own personal journey of training in Western medicine and later learning about yoga. Some concepts from ancient texts and teachings, including the *Yoga Sutras*, are presented. Ayurvedic medicine, which is an Eastern style of holistic medicine that has been practiced in India for thousands of years—sometimes called the sister science of yoga—will also be introduced. The chapter on ayurvedic medicine discusses the *doshas*, three groupings of bioenergetic traits that combine to characterize the physical, emotional, and mental characteristics of each individual. The determination of an individual's dosha type helps guide ayurvedic physicians and yoga therapists in choosing specific therapies to promote well-being.

Yogic teachings—including the energy centers (*chakras*), energy channels (*nadis*), and layers or aspects of individuals (*koshas*) —are discussed in the chapters that follow. Techniques regarding postures (asanas), breathing (pranayama), and meditation will be presented. The physiology of the autonomic nervous system, which works in the background to control many body functions, will be linked to various yoga practices. I also touch on some recent fascinating scientific studies that have demonstrated benefits of the practice of yoga and meditation. Case studies at the end of the book are intended to tie everything together as real-life examples of practical use.

I recommend that those who are new to these concepts try to avoid getting caught up in the terminology, and instead consider the broader ideas being presented. I place Sanskrit words in italics when introduced, except for some of the more common Sanskrit words such as asana (postures) and pranayama (breath). Sometimes, Latin words used in medical terminology or Sanskrit terms found in yoga can be intimidating when unfamiliar. I recommend that you keep reading and try to see the relationships presented, instead of trying to memorize unfamiliar terms. Think of this book as a "holistic" read rather than a textbook.

My hope is that you will find these subjects as fascinating as I do and find that the tools presented are practical for use in your own daily life. I admit that I was initially skeptical of some concepts such as the *chakras* when I first learned about them. But I have gradually merged my worldview and medical knowledge of anatomy and physiology with the teachings of yoga. This integration has allowed various concepts to make sense to me now. My hope is that this book will do the same for you.

A Brief History

The ancient practice of yoga, originating approximately 5000 years ago in India, started migrating to the Western world in the 19th century.[ii] Ralph Waldo Emerson, who had studied translations of ancient Hindu texts including the *Bhagavad Gita,* was influential in this migration. He published his essay "Nature" in 1836, which spearheaded the American Transcendentalist movement. His poem "Brahma" later appeared in the newly formed *Atlantic Monthly* in 1857, reflecting his concepts of Hindu spirituality.

Emerson heavily influenced Henry David Thoreau, who was perhaps the first American to consider himself a practicing yogi. Thoreau wrote *Walden* while living on land owned by Emerson. These two influential Transcendentalists favored individual exploration of spirituality, especially utilizing the presence of nature rather than religious dogma.

Perhaps the first person traditionally trained in India to introduce yoga to the West was Swami Vivekananda, a young monk from Kolkata (Calcutta). In 1894 he attended the World's Fair and the Parliament of the World's Religions in Chicago. A powerful speaker, he electrified audiences while speaking about yoga, Hinduism, and India. He continued on an influential tour of the US and published *Raja Yoga* in 1896, interpreting and translating from Sanskrit the teachings from Patanjali's *Yoga Sutras.*

Turning now to the history of Western medicine, the classic textbook *Gray's Anatomy* was first published in 1858, the work of Dr. Henry Gray and his coworker and illustrator Dr. Henry Vandyke Carter. A few years before, the Anatomy Act of 1832 had been passed in England. Prior to this, it was illegal to dissect any human bodies except for executed murderers. Now having legal access to corpses, these two talented men dedicated many hours to the cadaver lab. Dr. Carter helped with dissections and produced the meticulously accurate and beautiful illustrations. The book *Gray's Anatomy* was an instant best seller, and subsequent editions have been used by generations of medical students as an integral part of their training.

Dr. Gray unfortunately died from smallpox at the youthful age of 34. Dr. Carter, who was never given due credit or proper financial reward for his work on the book, left England to practice medicine in Mumbai (Bombay) with the Indian Medical Service. Dr. Carter represents an early example of Western and Eastern medicine co-mingling and sharing knowledge, including his profound expertise in anatomy. After 30 years he returned to England and died at the age of 65 from tuberculosis.

The fascinating Indra Devi, born in Russia in 1899 and originally named Eugenie V. Peterson, was influential in spreading yoga throughout the Western world. When she was a teen, she and her mother fled Russia for Berlin during the Bolshevik Revolution. In her twenties she moved to India, changing her name to Indra Devi for a successful career as a film star. In 1937 she stayed with the Maharaja and Maharini of Mysuru (Mysore) and met Sri Krishnamacharya, who ran a yoga school sponsored by the palace. She requested to be taught yoga, but initially was refused because she was both a Westerner and female. Yoga at that time had traditionally been considered a practice for men.

Eventually the Maharaja persuaded Sri Krishnamacharya to take Indra Devi as a student. Dedicating herself to the practice, in time she impressed Sri Krishnamacharya. He subsequently encouraged the multilingual Devi to go out into the world and spread the teachings of yoga. After a stint teaching in China, she introduced yoga to Hollywood around 1947 and taught many of the stars, including Gloria Swanson and Greta Garbo. She went on to travel and teach worldwide, as documented in Michelle Goldberg's fascinating *The Goddess Pose: The Audacious Life of Indra Devi, the Woman Who Helped Bring Yoga to the West.* Indra Devi died at the age of 102 in Argentina, where she was much beloved.

Another interesting and more controversial influence on yoga in the United States was Pierre Bernard. Born in Iowa in 1875, his birthname was Perry Arnold Baker. When he was a teenager living in Lincoln, Nebraska, he was introduced to tantric yoga by his neighbor. Baker embraced this style of yoga, studying and traveling with this mentor for years. Baker eventually changed his name to Pierre Bernard and opened a yoga school in New York City. Accused of misdeeds with a young female student in 1910, the notoriety caused him to leave the city and establish a country club style ashram on the Hudson River. He ran this lavish complex for years catering to the rich, including the Vanderbilts who helped bankroll him.

The Great Oom by Robert Love explores the enigmatic life of Pierre Bernard, who died in 1955. Bernard's story represents the intersection of capitalism, mysticism, celebrity, and tantric yoga. The sexual scandals also demonstrate his possible abuse of ethical responsibilities as a teacher. Bernard's story is a precursor of more recent episodes involving allegations of exploitation and sexual abuse by some gurus and senior teachers at certain schools or ashrams. Students should be cautioned to decide for themselves what practices and beliefs promote their own personal health and well-being. Blindly accepting instructions from a mentor as dogma may lead to unhealthy relationships, coercion, and traumatic experiences. Manipulating students from a position of power is unacceptable and certainly contradicts the true teachings of yoga.

Moving on in history, during the Vietnam war era and the rising social protests of the 1960's, yoga experienced a resurgence in popularity in the Western world. Exposure to the culture of India was fueled by the interest of the Beatles, the hippie era, and the music of Ravi Shankar. Young Americans and Europeans started traveling to India to study yoga with protegees of Sri Krishnamacharya and other gurus. In turn, these travelers have become some of the more famous senior yogis teaching worldwide today.

Spreading the Positive Benefits of Yoga

I have personally embraced incorporating yoga into my lifestyle for its physical health benefits. My relationship to stress has been transformed, and I am kinder and more content. Being mindful of the philosophical teachings has also improved me as a human being. I have learned to love and nurture myself, and in turn I am more loving to those around me.

I believe that each of us is a unique individual, yet we are all connected energetically. Our thoughts influence our attitudes, emotions, and actions toward those we are in contact with. In turn, other people's thoughts, emotions, and actions affect us too. These interactions can have a snowball effect, promoting anger and hostility for example, or they can promote kindness and compassion. By choosing more positive ways of thinking and attitudes in life, such as those taught in yoga, we tend to be more loving within ourselves and in our actions. This energetic effect produced by our attitude can rebound and positively benefit the world around us.

My body, mind, and soul treasure this precious gift of life with its ups and downs, unfolding moment by moment. I invite you to explore the teachings of yoga, then to integrate the practice of yoga into your lifestyle. You are likely to experience a more holistic sense of your body, mind, and spirit, leading to greater equanimity and ease. You potentially hold the power to not only improve your physical and mental health, but also to enrich your spirituality in profound ways.

Chapter Two:
A Physician's Perspective on Yoga

Yoga Sutras Meet *Gray's Anatomy*

Gray's Anatomy, as mentioned, is a classic textbook originally published in 1858. It has been widely used by students of anatomy, as I did in my graduate medical programs. The *Yoga Sutras* by Patanjali is a short book of aphorisms written somewhere between 500 BCE and 400 CE. The *Yoga Sutras* presents a concise overview of some of the traditional teachings of yoga that had been passed down through the ages. I include more about the *Yoga Sutras* in the next chapter. Both these texts have been influential to me and countless other students of anatomy and yoga.

My background as a healthcare professional has influenced my own unique outlook toward yoga, perceived largely through the lens of anatomy and physiology. My first real job was working as an orthopedic physician assistant (PA) for five years, which was a wonderful and challenging career. The practice I worked in was extremely busy with inpatient (hospital) rounds, emergency room care, and clinic responsibilities. In addition to learning about fracture care, arthritis, joint replacements, reading X-rays, and casting, I learned about the healing process.

Orthopedic issues or injuries can affect the whole body. It is not just one joint that is the problem: a hip or knee or back problem also affects the body elsewhere. The initial issue or injury may negatively influence your posture, the ability to perform various activities of daily living, and the ability to exercise for fitness. Thus, overall health may decline. Abnormal posture from an injury or arthritis places more stress on other joints in the body. Your fascia, or connective tissue, can "deform" and get stuck in this abnormal position over time. This cinching effect from poor posture by our connective tissue can create a vicious cycle, aggravating or even causing other orthopedic problems.

A patient's inability to do certain activities of daily life can cause a loss of independence as well as affect their relationships. Over time, the physical and mental stress of managing injuries and chronic pain often leads to a dependence on others for care of the home, driving, shopping, and personal hygiene. A patient may start to experience mental health issues including excessive anger, depression, and loss of self-esteem, which is likely to also be hard on the caregivers. In addition, pain control and dependency on pain prescriptions, along with their side-effects, can be negative contributing factors to the lifestyle, activity level, and mood changes in the patient. To summarize, in my job as a PA, I learned the initial injury or arthritic joint can affect many aspects of the patient's life: other parts of the body, the patient's activities and dependency on others, medications and their side-effects, lifestyle, and mental health. My exposure to this way of thinking about a patient holistically would influence my future choices in life.

Professionally, I eventually felt drawn to expand my knowledge and returned to school to study for a medical degree. Since I was more interested in working with the entire body rather than in a sub-specialty, I chose family practice for my residency training. Family practice often involves caring for several members of a family such as spouses, children, grandparents, and siblings. When I saw someone as a patient, I would often know what was going on with other family members too. These relationships, including the family's attitudes toward illness and each other, can influence the health of each individual. I saw that a variety of other factors—type of diet, activity level, prescription use, emotional and mental stress—all contribute to the development of illness and the ability of the patient to be resilient and recuperate.

My own life as a family practice physician was fulfilling, busy, and stressful. My family was growing, with the birth of three children over the next few years. As many readers know, juggling family life involving young children with a career is challenging. When the ballet studio that my girls attended started offering yoga for parents, I signed up and quickly became hooked. The immediate mental stress reduction as well as the physical workout really appealed to me.

I was fascinated by the effect of yoga compared to other forms of exercise I had practiced and wanted to learn more about it. However, my responsibilities as a physician and parent did not allow much free time to pursue this curiosity, other than attending classes. A few years later, thanks to my spouse's support, I was able to retire from my medical practice to be home for my children's important teenage years. As my kids started to become young adults, I decided to further my knowledge of yoga and took certification courses in yoga teacher training and yoga therapy. A whole new world opened to me about how to approach health and the human body.

Since then, I have expanded my yoga career to become a certified yoga therapist through the International Association of Yoga Therapists (IAYT). Yoga therapy is a relatively new profession in the United States. Yoga therapists typically work with either individuals or small groups with specific problems and common goals, using a variety of yoga tools to improve overall well-being. Some examples of therapeutically themed group classes are low-back issues, prenatal and postnatal care, cancer, cardiac rehab, and Parkinson's disease. Private one-on-one sessions for clients may include inpatient or outpatient referrals from healthcare practitioners. The individual client's specific needs and goals can be addressed in depth, often with the yoga therapist as a part of an integrative healthcare team.

I personally love sharing my knowledge and passion for yoga and healthcare by lecturing and giving workshops to medical students, residents, health professionals, yoga teachers, and students. Looking back on my life, my experience as a PA started my fascination with and appreciation for the human body in all its complexity. I am still awed at the body's physical powers of healing. Family practice reinforced the importance of holistic medicine in helping patients achieve optimal health, teaching me to look at the whole patient, rather than just addressing their chief complaint. My family practice experience mirrors the comprehensive approach of yoga and the ancient Indian system of ayurvedic medicine, which I learned about later in life.

Ayurvedic medicine considers the whole patient, including environment factors, and attempts to balance all the interdependent parts to achieve harmony. Yoga is one of the therapeutic tools often used in ayurvedic medicine. Yoga therapy utilizes the *pancha maya kosha* model, a concept of five layers or sheaths which comprise us as individuals. Briefly, these layers in individuals are the physical, energetic, emotional, mental, and spiritual selves. Though these five aspects or selves are considered subsets within us, each part affects the others.

Physical issues are intertwined with our ability to be active and energetic, which in turn influences our emotional, mental, and even spiritual state. The reverse is also true; mental or emotional problems affect our energy level and physical body. Attitudes affect outcomes, an example of a holistic approach. Ayurvedic medicine will be discussed more in Chapter Four.

The wisdom of yoga provides specific tools that are accessible to virtually everyone. I often wonder how my medical practice might have been different if I had been exposed to yoga earlier in my career. I would have had more tools in my repertoire to offer patients, and perhaps more patients would have been empowered to assume a partnership role in their healthcare. In my experience, the physician and patient working as a team inspires better results than does the physician assuming primary responsibility to "heal the patient." The old-fashioned paternalistic view of the physician-patient relationship is outdated, and healthcare is evolving into a partnership role. More responsibility taken by the patient can also help decrease the stress experienced by the healthcare provider. Professional burnout is a genuine issue in Western medicine. My prescription for burnout is to practice yoga, even if it is in very brief moments of time taken out throughout the day.

The Power of Stress

Stress is our physiological, mental, and emotional response to stressors or events in our lives. We all have stress; some is normal and can even be good for us, challenging our ability, adaptability, and coping skills. Stressors, the causes of stress, can vary in intensity from high to low, can be chronic and ongoing versus acute and short term, and can be actual versus perceived. There are distinct types of stressors, such as physical, environmental, mental, emotional, and spiritual. Some people cope better with stressors and are more resilient, perceiving less stress than their cohorts in similar situations. Some people even thrive on it, almost like an "adrenaline rush."

The body's response to perceived stressors impacts health, just as lifestyle and relationships do. A state of stress is reflected by a physiological reaction in the body. Higher cortisol and other "stress hormones" are produced, which in turn trigger a cascade effect. The physiological response of the body to chronic or high stress levels can affect the body on multiple levels, including inflammation in the cardiovascular system and impaired immune function. This inflammatory cascade triggered by chronic stress is thought to be one underlying factor in the development of multiple illnesses, including type 2 diabetes and heart disease. Unhealthy lifestyle habits—like smoking, being sedentary or overweight, and poor food choices—are other factors contributing to an underlying chronic inflammatory state. Trying to control the stress level, along with healthy food choices and exercise, can help reverse this process.

How can we learn to reduce tension as we respond to stressors in our lives? The physiological stress reaction sometimes feels like a whistling teapot that needs to release steam. How can we release this steam to prevent it from building up in our systems? Or better yet, how can we learn not to build up steam, in the form of chronic stress reactions, in the first place?

Herein lies the beauty of yoga. Yoga provides tools to better handle stressors and to decrease the chronic stress response in the body. I believe this ability to decrease stress, including lowering of circulating stress hormones, is the main reason yoga works for so many people. Techniques that help to decrease stress include using certain breathwork, the physical postures of yoga (asana), awareness, meditation, and cultivating kindness and compassion. Using these accessible tools, we can impact physical, mental, and spiritual health in a beneficial way. We can even learn to use specific techniques to decrease the stress response to whatever is happening in the present moment.

The autonomic nervous system (ANS) is responsible for the background physiological state of the body, typically without voluntary conscious control. The ANS traditionally had two main branches, the sympathetic and parasympathetic nervous systems. The enteric nervous system of the gut, which is discussed later, is now also thought of as a third branch of the ANS. The "fight or flight" stress response represents the sympathetic nervous system (SNS), and among other things produces a fast heart rate, high blood pressure, sweating, hypervigilance, and shunts blood away from the gut to the muscles. The SNS is the response of the body to stressors, both actual and perceived, readying the body to fight or flee. Conversely, the parasympathetic nervous system (PNS) cues the body to "rest and digest" by producing a lower blood pressure, slower heart rate, less muscle tension, mental relaxation, and shunts blood to the gut. The PNS also favors a healthy immune function. The SNS and PNS work together to help the body respond appropriately in any given moment to what life presents to us.

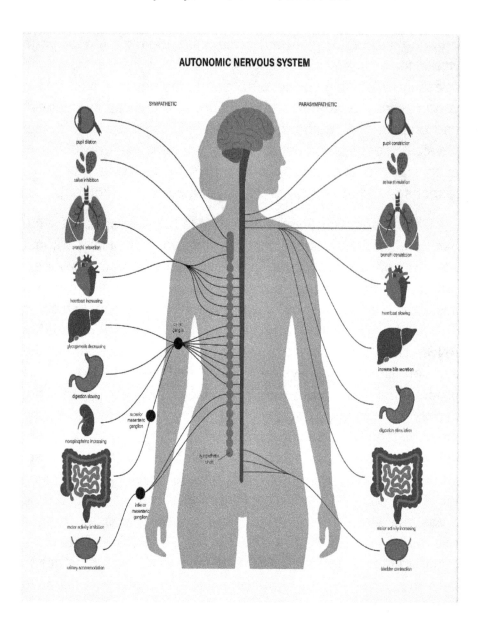

When you feel stress reactions of the SNS taking place in your body, such as anxiety and fast heart rate, you can use specific yogic styles of breathing (pranayama) to induce a calming PNS response, thereby counteracting your stressful "sympathetic storm." You can also learn to change your attitude and reaction to life stressors. Mindfulness helps you become more aware of the present and to respond to stressors in a calm helpful way, rather than to act impulsively or with a habitual stress response. Cultivating this yogic awareness or mindfulness in everyday life may eventually result in the stressors failing to produce a stress reaction at all. You may remain calm and unfazed. This desired goal requires commitment and practice but is attainable.

Sounds too good to be true? Please stay engaged and keep reading, and then *practice yoga.* Reading alone does not equal practice. Until you use the yoga tools yourself, the concepts of stress reduction and being more harmonious are just words, instead of being experienced by you, the individual practicing yoga.

Yoga as Integrative Medicine

Some of the popular styles of yoga practiced today leave out many of the ancient yogic concepts and instead focus mainly on the physical postures, asanas, as a form of exercise. Asana practice is extremely beneficial for developing the body-brain connection, such as interoception, and for other benefits. Interoception is being aware of sensations arising within the body, versus focusing on external sensations arising from the environment. But yoga encompasses so much more than the physical practices. Traditional teachings include behavioral guidelines for reducing suffering to self and others (the *yamas* and *niyamas*), breath techniques (pranayama), mindfulness (a Buddhist tradition), and meditation. These practices may be incorporated into your daily life, rather than just using them while you are on a yoga mat.

Western medicine tends to categorize illnesses into body systems, such as cardiovascular, respiratory, and endocrine systems. Even though underlying stressors and unhealthy lifestyles are acknowledged, the focus is on treating the part of the body that is "presenting" with the actual symptoms of the disease. Western medicine has an extensive repertoire of pharmaceuticals and procedures available for use that can be highly effective to treat symptoms, especially for acute issues.

However, when health professionals recommend lifestyle changes like diet and exercise, it is often a hard sell to get the patient to follow through. Patients tend to prefer a quick fix, such as a pill for high blood pressure. While pharmaceuticals can be effective, a pill is rather like putting a finger in the dike that represents the greater problem. High blood pressure is often a symptom of lifestyle, such as being overweight and sedentary, making poor food choices, and/or having chronic stress. Eating properly, controlling body weight, building up the physical body, and dealing with mental issues and stressors are more holistic goals to help get the blood pressure under control. The integrative lifestyle choices taught in yoga therapy can be influential as adjunct therapy for chronic conditions such as high blood pressure.

Rather than being separate approaches, yoga and Western medicine working together may complement each other to improve physical and mental health. An individual may be empowered to self-nurture, rather relying on the health professionals to "fix" them. This shouldering of responsibility by the individual to treat the precious body with respect can powerfully assist health professionals in caring for patients.

When health professionals understand and practice yoga themselves, it may influence patients to embrace their own lifestyle changes. Yoga as a recommendation from health professionals can be particularly helpful with chronic issues such as depression, adult-onset diabetes, high blood pressure, fibromyalgia, osteoarthritis, scoliosis, and chronic pain.[iii] Improvement in chronic illnesses may allow the healthcare professional to potentially wean patients off long-term use of medications such as those used for high cholesterol, high blood pressure, and pain control. This is especially relevant with the current problem of opioid overuse. Yoga is also a valuable preventive medicine tool to help maintain and prolong good health.

Physical bodies often reflect the story of what has happened in our lives. An example of the effects of stress on physical appearance is the aging of American presidents, comparing photos before and after serving their terms. Physical injuries, emotional and mental stress, diet, and physical fitness level all shape and mold us over time. Some people reflect health and confidence in their posture and affect, while others project fatigue, fear, depression, or anger. Habitual postural and movement patterns can cause certain muscle groups to become weak and "stuck" in either long or short positions due to sedentary or stressful lifestyles. Envision the common forward head position and the slouched posture of those who sit too much, and the hunched shoulders of the chronically stressed.

Yoga asana can help open and release these stuck muscles and fascial patterns. Incorporating teachings such as the *kleshas,* impediments to spiritual growth discussed in Chapter Five, can help release associated negative stressful patterns of thought.

Keeping an open mind about new concepts and evolving knowledge is important in both the modern medical field and in the practice of yoga. Ideas presented in this book are not set in stone. As we progress in our collective knowledge of these topics, some of the ideas here may evolve, prove to be incorrect, or need to be modified. One of my biggest challenges in drafting this book was that I am constantly learning and having new experiences. Inevitably, each time I reviewed the manuscript, I had learned something new, so I needed to make updates. I believe that the more you know, the more you realize there is so much to learn!

Importantly, yoga has also taught me to release my imagined control of the universe, welcome change, and move forward in a positive and hopeful direction. I realize that change is the only real constant in life and that perfection is elusive. Letting go of the idea of a perfect book has helped me stop revising and editing the manuscript and instead release the work for publication. I am proud of my effort, and, as Krishna advised Arjuna in the *Bhagavad Gita*, I am doing my best not to be attached to any particular outcome. The process of finalizing the book is a metaphor for moving on with my life, embracing change, releasing control and self-criticism, and removing the idea of perfection from my ego.

Each experience and person you encounter can give lessons in living. But you are your own most important teacher. Challenge yourself to stay open to new ideas and ways of thinking. Strive to choose what feels true to you at each moment. This wonderful life journey can truly be a blessing. Put forth the effort to be present in your own evolution towards a more contented union of body, mind, and spirit, which is the true goal of yoga.

Just as it is difficult to know where to start when instructing a new group of medical students about the vast knowledge of Western medicine, the same is true with the topic of yoga, which is as vast and far more ancient than modern medicine. In the next chapter, I focus on some ancient yogic texts, including Patanjali's *Yoga Sutras*, a guide to living a healthier, more compassionate, and fulfilling life.

Chapter Three:
Ancient Yoga Teachings and Texts

Yoga was traditionally passed down throughout the millennia from teacher to student via verbal instruction and memorization. The teachings originated in India more than five thousand years ago and were more spiritually focused compared to what yoga has evolved into today. Eventually the various schools of yoga philosophy transcribed the lessons into ancient Sanskrit texts that are the cornerstones of yoga. The *Vedas* are collections of various sacred Hindu scriptures from different time periods, dating as far back as 1500 BCE. It was believed that the scriptures were "received" teachings, that is, not authored by any one individual, having traditionally been taught over the generations orally. Since yoga originated in India, the Hindu religion plays a prominent historical part.

At the end of the *Vedas* are the Vedanta texts, several of which are the *Upanishads*, which discuss the concepts of *Atman* (individual soul) and *Brahman* (universal God). The spiritual philosophy contained in these texts is profound. The concepts of dualism and nondualism appear, including differing points of view within the various texts.[iv] Dualism, broadly speaking, refers to the individual soul and God as being separate entities. Conversely, nondualism, also called monism, refers to God as being within us, an inherent part of each one of us, rather than a separate entity. Vedanta ("the end, or culmination, of the *Vedas*") marks the beginning of the empowerment of the individual to connect directly with the divine rather than through the priestly Brahmins and their rituals. Some of these texts introduce the radical concept that liberation might be achieved by uniting

Atman (individual soul) with Brahman (ultimate reality). The *Kata Upanishad*, one of the Vedanta texts, contains the earliest use of the word "yoga" as we might understand it today. The *Bhagavad Gita* is also a Vedantic text, offering teachings of yoga related to how to live in the world.

I like to relate the concepts of dualism and nondualism to my own childhood religious instructions. I was brought up in the Catholic religion and was taught that God has three parts called the Holy Trinity, comprised of God the Father, the Son, and the Holy Spirit. As a child, when I prayed to the first two as entities, I thought of myself as separate from them, an example of dualism. God the Father was a strict older white man with a beard who could get angry and cause tragedies like Noah's flood. He turned people into pillars of salt and asked Abraham to sacrifice his own son. God the Father terrified me, which was at least part of the intention I believe, to make me act according to the Catholic doctrines. The Son, Jesus Christ, was wise, kind, and loving—not scary—but more tragic than the Father, as the depictions of the crucifixion constantly drove home. I felt guilty that he had suffered and died for our sins. When I prayed to God the Father or God the Son, I thought of them as separate entities from myself, or dualistic concepts.

As a child, my personal favorite from the Holy Trinity was the Holy Spirit, who could commune with me in the form of a white dove. How cool to have this beautiful white bird magically enter and mingle with my soul! The Holy Spirit was like talking to a friend inside of me who did not make me feel scared or guilty. Rather than an intimidating male figure, the Holy Spirit was more like a guardian angel, always accessible and nurturing to me as a child. My concept of the Holy Spirit served as a precursor to the appeal of yoga's nondualist teachings that I encountered many years later as an adult. The idea of being able to look within myself to find my inner wisdom, and the feeling that I am intermingled with God, is more appealing to me than thinking of God as some separate entity.

My personal adult concept of nondualism or monism implies that the spirit (*Atman*) within is part of the universal God (*Brahman*), and all is interconnected. This spirit or life force exists in each one of us and is present throughout the universe. My internal microcosm—down to the cellular, molecular, and atomic level—is energetically connected with the immense macrocosm of the universe outside of my physical body. In an oversimplistic model, individuals and the universe alike are made up of photons, stardust, and atoms with huge areas of empty space linking everything. Yet I am inherently valued and loved by a presence larger than myself, just as each of my body cells is valued and loved by me. My tiny source of individual energy does not compare with the universe, the immense energy of God, which is beyond my comprehension. To be valued and loved by this Immensity is overwhelmingly comforting to me.

The *Vedas*, the *Upanishads*, and the *Bhagavad Gita*

Returning to the subject of ancient texts, transcriptions of surviving texts of the *Vedas* were originally translated into Persian in about the 15th century and into Latin, English, and German in the 1800s. These teachings were embraced by Western philosophers, poets, and scholars including Ralph Waldo Emerson, Henry David Thoreau, Walt Whitman, W.B. Yeats, and T.S. Eliot.[v] Among these historically important texts is the *Bhagavad Gita*.

"I have made the Bhagwad Gita as the main source of my inspiration and guide for the purpose of scientific investigations and formation of my theories."

~ Albert Einstein

The *Bhagavad Gita* was probably composed about 200 BCE. It is a part of the *Mahabharata*, an important epic poem from ancient India. The *Bhagavad Gita* describes the struggle of a great warrior named Arjuna. He has a crisis of consciousness when confronted with the prospect of killing relatives and loved ones who are on opposing sides in a great battle. His charioteer is Krishna, an avatar or reincarnation of Vishnu, who is one of the Hindu deities. Arjuna and Krishna have a prolonged philosophical discussion that includes the concepts of *dharma* (duty), different spiritual paths to the divine, the relationship between *Atman* and *Brahman*, and release from ignorance and suffering. The last of these important yogic concepts I discuss in a later chapter on the *kleshas* (causes of pain and suffering). The value of the *Bhagavad Gita* and other Vedic texts is demonstrated by the fact that they have survived thousands of years and still are relevant to the human condition. I encourage you to explore a good translation, as have many scholars throughout the centuries.

Yoga Sutras

The *Yoga Sutras* by Patanjali is a collection of aphorisms or sutras linking yogic concepts. It was compiled somewhere between 500 BCE to 400 CE. The *Yoga Sutras* is one of the oldest surviving written texts concerning the teachings of what is known as *Raja* (kingly) yoga and the eightfold path.[vi] Unification of body-mind-spirit, release from the cycles of pain and suffering, and achieving enlightenment towards a state of bliss are the goals of Raja yoga. The *Yoga Sutras* has had a resurgence in popularity as a teaching tool for yoga training programs and as a concise reference for some of the teachings of yoga. Contrary to our current concept of yoga, the book does not include any physical postures, except for the mention of sitting comfortably with both ease and strength for meditation.

Important concepts include choosing an honorable lifestyle and coming in touch with the true inner self or *Atman*. *Atman* can be thought of as the soul, spirit, or life force. This eternal self exists before and after our mortal life and is the only truly permanent part of us. Ignorance of this fact is the basic cause of most pain and suffering. We get caught up in our ego, bodies, and this material world, including desires/attachments and aversions/fears. The *Yoga Sutras* deal with steps to get past this ignorance and strive towards a more meaningful and fulfilled life.

These steps are called the eightfold path, listed below with discussion following. The eightfold path as written in the *Yoga Sutras* is subject to translational differences from the original Sanskrit, as well as subject to individual interpretations, especially in view of how our society has evolved over the past two thousand years. However, these methods outlined in the eightfold path are still relevant today for improving physical, mental, and spiritual health. Note that my personal interpretation of these teachings may differ from that of others. I also want to clarify that the eightfold path of yoga is different from the eightfold path of Buddhism, though both are worthy teachings.

1. *Yamas*...social restraints

   a) *Ahimsa*...non-violence
   b) *Satya*...truthfulness
   c) *Asteya*...non-stealing
   d) *Aparigraha*...non-grasping
   e) *Brahmacarya*...sensual restraint and moderate lifestyle

2. *Niyamas*...personal observances

   a) *Saucha*...cleanliness
   b) *Santosha*...contentment
   c) *Tapas*...effort
   d) *Svadhyaya*...self-study
   e) *Ishvara pranidhana*...surrender to and contemplation of the spiritual divine

3. *Asana*...postures

4. *Pranayama*...breath

5. *Pratyahara*...withdrawal of the senses

6. *Dharana*...concentration

7. *Dhyana*...contemplation

8. *Samadhi*...bliss

The *Yamas*

The *yamas*, five rules or restraints, are individual disciplines or practices to guide proper behavior in society. The first *yama*, *ahimsa*, broadly translates as "do no harm," which is similar to the Hippocratic Oath in medicine. Practicing a compassionate, kind, and nurturing attitude towards ourselves, others, and mother earth represents *ahimsa*. *Ahimsa* is the basis for why many yogis are vegetarians, choosing foods that are not only healthy for them, but also take less of the earth's resources to produce or deliver. Taking responsibility to do no harm to the environment diminishes our carbon footprint. Learning to be good to ourselves both physically and mentally and letting go of the self-criticism and judgment, which is often subconsciously projected onto others, also represents *ahimsa*.

The second *yama* is *satya,* or truthfulness. I have found that telling the truth makes life simpler; untruths are burdens that weigh down the soul. In addition to not speaking outright lies, trying to avoid telling untruths about life's potentials is part of this *yama*. It can be liberating to reject the "I can't" and "you don't" words and thoughts that can be subtle falsehoods, though probably unintentional. Having an open mind to life's possibilities for ourselves and others is important, rather than imposing negativity with limitations. This *yama* encourages us to be practical yet brave and positive in pursuing goals.

Asteya means non-stealing, which can be interpreted concretely to physical objects, but also extended to not stealing other people's joy or positivity. Coming home after an exhausting day of work can tempt us to "take it out" on loved ones and to bring them down to our fatigue level or bad mood. Recognizing this tendency can help us learn to reject this practice. Instead of stealing other's good moods, we can be open to their joyfulness. Positivity instead of negativity then becomes contagious and can bounce back to us.

Brahmacharya is translated as following God or practicing sensual restraint, using different connotations. This *yama* implies a moderation in lifestyle, including restraint from excessive transient sensory pleasures. TV and other social media show how obsessed our culture is with sex and food, as well as youth and physical beauty. *Brahmacharya* encourages us to turn inward to find joy, instead of being dominated excessively by the senses. Ancient sages embraced this practice by becoming celibate hermits, leaving their families behind to pursue their spiritual quests. Practicing *brahmacharya* by restraining impulsive sexual pleasures may help prevent negative long-term consequences, such as hurting others. Many lives would be simpler if we followed this advice, avoiding wounding loved ones. Children are often innocent victims of infidelity that can threaten family units. The sensory pleasure is only transient, but the wounded feelings and repercussions can be long term.

"Do not look for rest in any pleasure, because you were not created for pleasure: you were created for joy. And if you do not know the difference between pleasure and joy you have not yet begun to live"

~ Thomas Merton

Aparigraha, or non-grasping, the final *yama*, teaches us to avoid hoarding or lusting after more possessions, money, power, or fame. This term can also be applied to continually grasping at goals, and never being satisfied or content (*santosha)* unless we "make it" to some elusive goal. For some people, this struggle is never ending, and satisfaction is never achieved. Abiding by this *yama* includes learning to be content with our present situation, perhaps living in simpler surroundings, and focusing more on effort rather than goals. True self-worth should not be dependent on physical possessions, accolades, looks, or a massaged ego.

The *Niyamas*

The *Niyamas* are five observances practiced by an individual, or how one behaves when other people are not necessarily watching. The first *niyama*, *saucha*, means cleanliness of the body as well as the mind. *Saucha* involves keeping the body physically clean and choosing healthy foods and habits. To me, it also includes striving for positive versus negative thoughts and mental images. Over-exposure to frightening, gruesome, or brutal images and thoughts can form patterns in the brain that may replay and become troublesome. If we control our exposure, we may experience less stress and become more serene. We can still be aware of what is happening in the world without repetitively reinforcing those images and distressing the mind. Consider staying informed, then turn off media that tends to constantly play shocking news. Choose exposure to something positive instead of ruminating in negativity.

Tapas is applying effort towards goals, duties, and desires, including becoming a more spiritually fulfilled and knowledgeable being. Instead of giving in to sloth and stagnation, *tapas* allows us to grow and learn instead, while being respectful of the need for rest and recuperation periods. *Tapas* is a wonderful tool for bettering ourselves if applied to worthy goals. I often drew on this concept of effort when working on this book.

Tapas is balanced by *santosha,* or contentment. Even while putting forth effort, learn to be content with the activity of the present moment. The effort is the important thing, not the goal itself. *Tapas* allows life to unfold as we try to live up to our best potential, while *santosha* allows us not to fret about the outcome. In the process, perhaps another path or a new goal will open.

The *yama aparigraha* (non-grasping) can be applied here as well. *Santosha* also applies to being content with others, rather than trying to change them into our concept of what they should be.

Self-study, *svadhyaya,* is the next *niyama* and is a lifelong process. We really are our own best teachers. Each of us has a unique collection of experiences, memories, thoughts, and deeds. Admitting mistakes and unhealthy habits helps us make better choices next time. Mistakes build wisdom if we can learn to let go of the past instead of obsessing about it. *Svadhyaya* allows us to contemplate, make more thoughtful choices, and be more aware of the consequences of future actions.

"The organic gardener does not think of throwing away the garbage. She knows that she needs the garbage. She is capable of transforming the garbage into compost, so that the compost can turn into lettuce, cucumber, radishes, and flowers again...With the energy of mindfulness, you can look into the garbage and say: I am not afraid. I am capable of transforming the garbage back into love."

~ Thich Nhat Hanh

Svadhyaya can also help with difficult choices by noticing what the heart center is feeling. When faced with a dilemma, imagine going down both paths and see how the heart feels emotionally in the two different scenarios. Recognizing which choice makes the heart feel open and free, rather than constricted and closed, may help guide problematic decisions.

Ishvara pranidhana is contemplation of and surrender to the universe or God. To me, "surrender to the universe" means to release the idea that I am responsible for, or in control of, everything around me. Contemplation on God has different connotations to many people. Terms such as Brahma, Allah, the eternal life force, or universal cosmic energy may be substituted. Each individual's personal beliefs are not the only valid beliefs and should not be forced on other people. While open communication is helpful, attempts to overly control the world and those around us can lead to frustration and resentment. Nor are we as individuals responsible for all the world's woes, which would be overwhelming. *Ishvara pranidhana* allows us to accept that we are not the center of the universe. We should strive to help improve the world around us, without shouldering all the world's suffering.

Using all the *yamas* and *niyamas* allows us to explore our morality, mortality, and spirituality. This exploration may ultimately lead to facing death with dignity and curiosity rather than fear. People close to death care about love and relationships with others, not portfolios or fancy cars. Choosing love and kindness as our primary motivating force may be the most important goal in this mortal life. We should not wait until our deathbed to come to this realization. Accepting our own mortality can free us to treasure the present moments and savor each day more fully.

Asana

The third step in the eightfold path, following the *yamas* and *niyamas*, is asana, or the physical postures. A later chapter is devoted to diverse types of asanas in more detail. Asana is probably what most people think of when they consider yoga, but the only asana Patanjali mentions in the *Yoga Sutras* is being able to sit in a comfortable position for meditation. Since most people in modern society are conditioned to sitting on chairs, sitting on the ground or floor may be one of the more difficult asanas for beginners. There are several ways to modify this position, such as elevating the hips by sitting on a bolster. With practice, the spine becomes long and strong and the hips will open enough to sit more comfortably on the floor. Sitting on a chair with the spine upright is also a viable alternative for many people. To be still in the sitting position is beneficial for meditation. One is less likely to fall asleep, and the erect supportive spine gives a unique energy to the meditation. However, you can meditate in any position such as lying down, walking, or even while doing activities.

The concept of emphasizing the body in yoga with various asanas or postures as a form of exercise is relatively new in the history of yoga. Yoga postures perhaps first appeared in a book written about the 15th century, *The Hatha Yoga Pradipika,*[viii] which showed several different postures besides sitting. In the 1920s in British colonial India, a yoga teacher and scholar named Tirumalai Krishnamacharya popularized physical *hatha* yoga, incorporating European gymnastic components and elements of wrestling into asana practice. Krishnamacharya became one of the most influential figures in modern yoga. He was trying to bring the practice of yoga back to the people of colonial India, and this physical practice was an eye-catching advertisement. Eventually he gained the financial support of the Maharaja of Mysuru (Mysore) and opened Mysuru (Mysore) school of yoga. Krishnamacharya subsequently trained many influential yoga teachers, including B. K. S. Iyengar, Pattabhi Jois, T. K. V. Desikachar (Krishnamacharya's own son), and Indra Devi, all of whom in turn trained many of our current senior yoga teachers in the West today.[ix] Krishnamacharya is considered by some to be the father of modern *hatha* yoga, with its emphasis on asana.

Asana has many powerful beneficial effects on the body. Postures are best done initially under guidance from a good teacher, so alignment and safety principles are followed. Asana becomes a powerful tool to connect the body and the mind. All the concepts of the *yamas* and *niyamas* can be incorporated into asana practice, using mindful awareness as one progresses along the yogic path.

Pranayama

The study of the breath, pranayama (discussed in Chapter Six), is one of the most powerful tools in yoga and is available to virtually everyone, regardless of physical abilities. Pranayama practices give us the ability to affect our physiological states. Pranayama can be simple yet complex, and as a contemplative practice no two observations of the breath are ever exactly alike. Distinct styles of breath affect the autonomic nervous system (ANS), including the sympathetic nervous system (SNS) and parasympathetic nervous system (PNS), and can influence the neuro-endocrine system including release of hormones. The effect on the body and mind is to produce either an activating or a relaxing effect, or a balance of the two, depending upon the style of breath chosen and the goal.

The final four steps of the eightfold path involve varying degrees of meditation. They are discussed briefly below and in more depth in Chapter Nine.

Pratyahara

Pratyahara refers to withdrawal of the physical senses. One chooses an object of awareness to focus on and tries to prevent the distractions of the physical senses from interfering with this focus. Examples include focusing awareness on a certain body part during asana, on the breath with pranayama, or even on one sensation such as hearing. *Pratyahara* takes discipline and practice and can be equated with asana of the mind. Just as one can master a physical posture with practice, so can we learn to control the senses. The simplest way to start this practice is to shut the eyes, preventing visual distractions. Eventually other physical input or sensations can be observed and let go, turning the awareness to the subject of choice.

Dharana

Dharana (concentration) can be thought of as withdrawal from distracting thoughts, images, memories, or other unwanted mental functioning. Withdrawal of the physical senses, *pratyahara*, is taken to a deeper mental level. One method is to take the awareness to one or two subjects of choice to concentrate on. We are attempting to avoid being distracted—at least not for long—by either our senses or our thoughts, but instead to refocus and concentrate on the object of meditation.

Dhyana

Dhyana is uninterrupted effortless *dharana*, in which we are not distracted by the physical senses or thoughts. Rather than having to resist distractions and refocus the concentration, we move into a more contemplative mode in which awareness flows uninterrupted. We move from a state of doing to a state of being.

If we use the breath as the focus, we are intimately riding the breath without being distracted. Thoughts are not elsewhere. If you have ever become totally immersed in a project, book, or action so intently that you lose track of time and place, then you have at least partially experienced this state.

Samadhi

Dhyana, uninterrupted focus, or contemplation, then transforms into a deeper state of meditation, *samadhi,* in which you merge with the subject of your focus and become one with it. If the focal choice is the breath, you become your breath with nothing else occupying the mind. The observer and the observed become one. You lose your sense of I-ness or ego and are totally immersed in the moments of union with the object of contemplation. The state of samadhi is difficult to describe in words.

To me, a deeper way to conceive of *samadhi* is the process of merging individual awareness with the source of awareness itself. That deepest part of me, not the physical body, but the spirit, is my only true constant observer. In deep meditation, I move towards merging with and embracing this spiritual self. I think of this self as beneficent, joyful, wise; watching and waiting to embrace me back. When saints have described profound contemplative prayer as a union with God, I think of *samadhi.*

One of my favorite quotes is by Pierre Teilhard de Chardin. "We are not human beings having a spiritual experience; we are spiritual beings having a human experience." The soul has been present observing life's entire existence, and now the whole of our attention is turned onto the soul or life force. The soul, the constant background observer of life, is now being observed by unwavering awareness. The observer (soul/spirit/*Atman*) becomes the observed and rises to merge with the mortal self.

When I use breath as my initial focus, I like to think of a saying by B. K. S. Iyengar, a well-known *hatha* yoga teacher in India who taught so many Westerners and lived to the age of 95. To paraphrase him, the inhale is the soul rising up to meet the mortal body, and the exhale is the soul surrendering to the universe. What a wonderful path to *samadhi*. Typically, for me, *samadhi* is a brief transient experience if it happens at all. Be careful not to grasp for *samadhi*, but let the meditation unfold and be content with the present moment as it is happening. The more one grasps, the more evasive it is. Meditation is a practice. Rather than just being something taught or described, meditation is meant to be an experience.

To summarize, in this chapter I have presented a brief outline of the eightfold path. Some of the other important teachings in the *Yoga Sutras* will be discussed in further chapters. What do all these teachings have to do with Western medicine? If yoga is recommended to and embraced by an individual, enhanced by learning, good teachers, and self-study (*svadhyaya),* remarkable lifestyle changes may occur. The practice of yoga is like empowering yourself to become your own physical trainer, counselor, and spiritual mentor. The eightfold path does not have to be followed in any particular order. In the beginning you are taking baby steps to start what may become a lifelong journey. Those steps may include pursuing knowledge such as reading this book, asana practice on the yoga mat, adopting healthy lifestyle habits, practicing kindness and compassion, and/or attending to your spirituality.

Chapter Four:
Ayurvedic Medicine and the Doshas

Author's Disclaimer: I am not an ayurvedic physician or practitioner, and what I present and discuss is my understanding from my individual studies. You should consult an ayurvedic practitioner or text for more complete information. Always follow your own healthcare professional's recommendations for your medical care. Consultation should be done before making any changes in your diet, activity, or lifestyle. The information presented here is not meant to be medical advice or a substitute for your healthcare provider's expertise and recommendations. I do encourage you to be an advocate and partner with your provider in your own health care.

Ayurvedic medicine is an ancient form of holistic medicine originating in India, probably more than 5000 years old. It is based on the concept of three different sets of characteristics known as *doshas.* These three doshas, named pitta, kapha, and vata, each have different energetic properties, or qualities, which combine to produce the physical, mental, and personality traits of each individual. One dosha is typically more dominant in the individual. Characteristics of the different doshas can be compared to your genetic code, which affects your physical traits, personality, and temperament. The predominant dosha type of your physical body does not necessarily match the dosha type of your mental self or temperament.

Ideally, your dosha type is determined by consulting an ayurvedic physician who does various assessments. However, numerous tests or quizzes are available online to help approximate your ratio of the three doshas, though you lose the advantage of the physical exam and expertise of the ayurvedic physician. If you take a dosha quiz yourself, it may be helpful to ask someone close to you to also fill it out with you in mind. Then you can see if your own perception of your characteristics matches how another person perceives you. These tests will show the percentage of each of the three doshas that comprises your makeup, or your "baseline" dosha ratio.

According to ayurvedic medicine, you are in balance when you maintain your innate normal baseline dosha ratio. When life is on an even keel and nothing is rocking the boat, your doshas are usually in balance. But if the energetic effect of one of the doshas either rises (usually, but not necessarily your dominant dosha) or falls from the constitutional ratio, you become out of balance. As we will see, the seasons, environment, diet, and stage of life all affect the doshas. Unbalanced doshas are usually due to some type of stressor or disturbance. If not restored to balance, the result may escalate to develop symptoms or diseases.[x]

Ayurvedic medicine addresses these disturbances by using modalities such as diet, herbs, minerals, yoga, exercise, meditation, cleansing techniques, and surgery. The treatments are directed towards decreasing the dosha whose qualities have become too domineering and are disturbing your harmony. There are specific ways of treating each dosha to calm it down, the goal being to return to your normal preset balanced ratio of doshas.

Each of the doshas is represented by certain combinations of the elements of earth, water, fire, air, and space (ether), as shown in the figure below. The characteristics of these combinations, such as heaviness versus lightness, coolness versus heat, movement versus stillness, and moisture versus dryness, form the doshas. For example, earth, which is heavy, still, cool, and moist is a component of the kapha dosha, in which people tend to have a sturdy build and cool, moist skin. The chakras, discussed later in Chapter six, also have correlations with the elements.

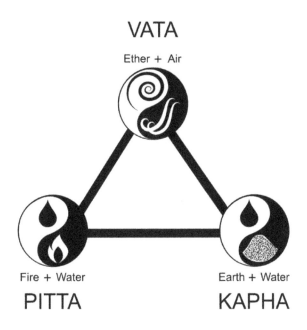

VATA

Ether + Air

Fire + Water
PITTA

Earth + Water
KAPHA

The following chart summarizes the doshas, including the associated elements, qualities, characteristics, symptoms when rising, and treatments for excess kapha, pitta, and vata. "Symptoms when rising" refers to situations when the effects of one dosha, usually your most prevalent one, grow and can become overpowering.

Dosha	kapha	pitta	vata
Elements	Earth and water	Water and fire	Air and ether/space
Qualities	Cool and moist	Moist and warm	Dry and cool
Characteristics	Strong, sturdy build, good endurance, faithful, loving, good memory but slower to grasp concepts, harder to get moving, cool and moist skin	Medium build, active, competitive, intelligent, ambitious, driven, warm and moist skin, ruddy complexion	Thin build, quick at grasping concepts but poorer memory, prefer movement physically and mentally, dry and thin skin
Symptoms/Seasons when "rising"	Weight gain, lethargy, depression, increased mucous production, increase in the late winter and spring	Overheating, hot and sweaty, anger, difficulty falling asleep, irritability, high blood pressure, heartburn, summer can aggravate	Anxious, weight loss, constipation, wake in middle of the night, coldness, cannot focus, restless, increases in the fall
Treatments	Diet: avoid carbohydrates, encourage warm, dry foods such as roasted vegetables Asana: needs active moving workout to burn energy and get moving Environment: dry warm such as desert to counter cool and moist qualities	Diet: avoid hot spicy foods and caffeine; better cool, dry, raw fruits and veggies Asana: perhaps a brief active workout then a slow practice to cool and relax Environment: cool and dry such as high altitudes to counter heat and moisture	Diet: avoid raw, cold, dry foods; use warm, moist such as stews and carbs Asana: grounding, such as slower paced or restorative practice Environment: warm and moist such as the tropics to counter cold and dry

Each dosha is also represented by five subdivisions of bodily functions and their corresponding locations in the body. While I will mention these, an ayurvedic text should be consulted for more detail.[xi] Health professionals and yoga therapists might find these subdivisions interesting because of some correlation with the Western medicine subspecialties. I suggest that you avoid getting bogged down in the names of the subdivisions; it is the relationships that are interesting.

The Kapha Dosha

The kapha dosha is composed of earth (coolness, heaviness, and stability) and water (lubrication, fluidity, moistness) properties and is represented by a body type that is strong and sturdy with moist cool skin, large attractive eyes, and full lips. Hair is thick and lustrous. When in balance, these individuals are loyal, loving, and strong steady workers with good memories. The chest and upper stomach are important physical sites for kapha.

When kapha is out of balance, obesity, inertia, and diseases with excess mucus, like sinus and respiratory congestion, can result. Personality traits such as greediness, hoarding, and attachment are other signs of excess kapha. In the Western medical system, metabolic syndrome—which includes obesity, high blood sugar, high triglycerides, low HDL (good cholesterol), and high blood pressure—could be thought of as excess kapha. Metabolic syndrome can progress to more serious problems like type two diabetes and cardiovascular disease. Low carbohydrate diets help counter the above components of metabolic syndrome, an example being the American Diabetic Association (ADA) diet. This correlates with the low carbohydrate diets used in ayurvedic medicine for excess kapha symptoms such as weight gain. Both Western and ayurvedic medicine recommend activity and exercise to counteract metabolic syndrome and excess kapha. Excess kapha symptoms tend to rise in the late winter and early spring when the weather is moist and cool. These seasons are often associated with being more sedentary and gaining weight.

Yoga asanas and breathing techniques that activate and energize the body are used to counterbalance excess kapha. People with body types subject to kapha imbalances need to get moving to treat their tendency towards inertia and weight gain. Diets that take more energy to digest, such as spicy foods and raw vegetables, can be helpful. Avoiding high-caloric and high-carbohydrate foods to decrease the kapha quality of heaviness is a key dietary treatment. Predominantly kapha types do best in warm dry localities, such as a desert, to counteract their moist, cool qualities.

Kapha is subdivided into five locations or functions in the body, as shown in the image below. Remember that kapha is represented by water and earth, so think about a combination of fluids, strength, and stability. The first subdivision, *kledaka*, is in the upper stomach and starts the initial breakdown of food by churning and liquifying solids into a thick substance called *chyme*. Gastric acid can be thought of as the liquid component representing kapha in the stomach. The second subdivision is known as *avakambhaka*, found in the chest, heart, and lungs, and represents the strength of the muscular pumping heart and lubrication of the respiratory mucosa. *Tarpaka*, the third subdivision, is in the head and spinal cord, with cerebrospinal fluid hydrating and cushioning the brain and spinal cord, representing mental calmness and stability. The fourth subdivision, *bodhaka*, located in the mouth and tongue, provides lubrication for both taste and salivation. Finally, *shleshaka* represents the lubrication of the joints by synovial fluid.[xii]

One can see how these subdivisions start to sound more like Western medicine's emphasis on subspecialties. *Kledaka* in the upper gut would be considered the realm of a gastroenterologist. In *avakambhaka*, the heart and lungs are covered by cardiology and pulmonary specialists. The head and spinal cord regions of *tarpaka* utilize neurology and psychology. *Bodhaka's* mouth and tongue falls under otolaryngology (ENT). Finally, in *shleshaka* the joints are in a rheumatologist and orthopedic surgeon's specialty. We shall see the other doshas also have body regions where their characteristics are prominent and can be correlated with Western medicines specialties.

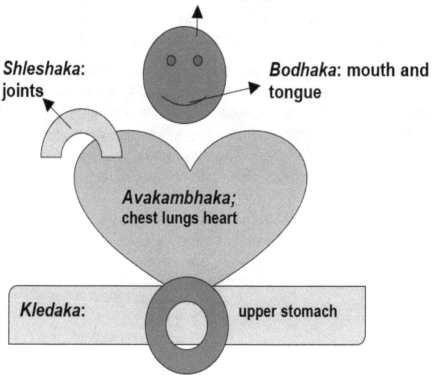

Kapha Dosha Sites

The Pitta Dosha

The pitta dosha is composed of fire and water properties. People with a pitta-dominant constitution are often ambitious with lots of drive and energy. Typical body build is of average size and musculature, with warm, moist skin prone to sweating and sunburn. Hair may be reddish or fair and is usually fine. Eyes can have an intense gaze. Pitta types are usually intelligent and confident. The upper gastrointestinal (GI) tract, *pachaka*, is the dominant site for this dosha. Transmutation, the act of changing one substance into a different form, is represented by pitta's digestive fire in the upper GI tract. Hence, the process of absorbing food and turning it into energy is an important characteristic of the pitta dosha. While the upper stomach was under kapha's domain with the churning and acid breakdown of food, pitta transforms those food particles into energy for cell use.[xiv]

This digestive fire is like a campfire. We do not want it too hot, turning into an uncontrolled blaze, like ulcers represent. Nor do we want it to go out by overeating, being unable to stoke the fire alive again, and food just sits undigested in our stomach. The same can be said of the energy levels in our body. Too much agitation on one hand, versus slothfulness on the other, represent extreme ranges of energy levels. Although all three doshas affect our energy levels, pitta importantly does so by transforming food into energy for the body. The eyes and vision are also important sites for pitta, as the light energy striking the retina stimulates the visual brain receptors. Transforming visual input into perception, thought, intelligence, and then action is an example of transmutation of energy.

When pitta is in excess, there may be too much heat and intensity in the body. In terms of Western medicine, Type A personalities with high blood pressure, ulcers, GERD (heartburn), gallbladder problems, and anger-control issues are often influenced by excess pitta. The hypervigilant component of PTSD could be included as a symptom of excess pitta in the mind. Problems initiating sleep and overheating are other symptoms. Remember, not just pitta dominant people can experience these symptoms. A predominantly vata or kapha dosha may also have episodes in life which cause their pitta components to rise, resulting in symptoms such as anger, difficulty getting to sleep, and heartburn.

Asana practice to help overactive pitta might include some initially vigorous exercise to burn off the excess energy, followed by a more important calming practice such as restorative yoga to produce coolness. For example, starting with a moving flow type yoga may rid the body and mind of extra energy and restlessness. Then the more important part of the asana practice would be cooling and relaxing, such as laying on the floor and stretching while supported by bolsters. Dietary recommendations might include decreasing caffeine, alcohol, and the spiciness of the diet, just as Western medicine does for heartburn and ulcers. Cooling foods like salads, raw fruits, and vegetables are helpful.

Closing the eyes, an example of *pratyahara* (withdrawal of the senses), can be helpful for overactive pitta by providing a respite from visual input. Humans are primarily visual beings. Sight activates your brain to transform light striking the retina into impressions and thoughts. Taking a visual time-out can calm the competitiveness in pittas that may be fueled by the sense of vision, such as comparison with others in a yoga class. Summer heat and humidity are also hard on those with a dominance of pitta, who tend to do better in cool, dry environments. Shielding the skin and eyes from UV light also decreases "fire" exposure from the sun and helps prevent eye damage and skin cancer. Pittas tend to be redheads or fair complexioned which may increase their risk of sun damage. Meditation while closing the eyes and visualizing a calm, cool place, such as a high-altitude mountaintop, can be soothing for excess pitta. Learning to open the heart to positive emotions such as gratitude, compassion, and love may be transformative for rising pitta, counterbalancing the tendency for dominating and judging others, competitiveness, and jealousy.

Pachaka, found in the upper GI tract, is the most important site of pitta, harboring the digestive fire as discussed above. *Alochaka*, responsible for vision, transforms visual input into thought. Other pitta subdivisions include *ranjaka* in the liver, gallbladder, and spleen, responsible for the color in stool and red blood cell production. *Sadhaka*, in the heart, represents how absorbing experiences affect emotions and the mental state. We tend to feel our emotions in our heart area, as lots of our colloquialisms demonstrate like "my heart leapt for joy" and "he/she broke my heart." The emotional heart transforms experiences into emotions like joy or sadness, and feelings like love or hate. When people are asked to point to themselves, they usually indicate the heart area, indicating how intensely important this area is to our sense of being. The last location of pitta is *bharajaka* in the skin, giving luster, color, and warmth.[xv]

These locations can again be correlated with the Western medical specialties. Gastroenterology deals with *pachaka* in the upper GI tract as well as *ranjaka* sites in the liver, gall bladder, and stool. Hematology also treats *ranjaka* sites corresponding with red blood cells production, including the spleen. Ophthalmology deals with *alochaka* in the eyes. *Sadhaka* in the heart is under the domain of cardiology and psychiatry, with the effect on our emotions and mood. *Bharajaka* in the skin falls under dermatology.

Many illnesses can be thought of as too much "heat" in the body, representing an out-of-control pitta dosha and excessive stimulation of the sympathetic nervous system (SNS). When the SNS kicks in, pupils dilate, the heart races, blood pressure rises, breathing changes, blood is pumped to our muscles, and our skin flushes and sweats. We are more alert and may experience anxiety. Hopefully, this is a transient state once the stressor is removed. But some people, particularly pittas, can be in a more chronic state of SNS dominance. They have a lot of energy and drive which may be beneficial, but conversely can also find it difficult to relax and unwind. This state of excess energy may result in chronic conditions like hypertension (high blood pressure) which can lead to heart disease and strokes. Excessive mental or emotional stress can be thought of as overstimulation, like an engine running too hot, which can permeate the physiology. This stimulation, unresolved, can cause physiological symptoms like high blood pressure, ulcers, insomnia, and skin diseases, representing inflammation in the body. Many chronic illnesses in Western medicine are thought to have an inflammatory basis. As discussed earlier, by calming a chronic stress response, you may improve your overall physical and mental health. In general, pittas benefit from calming the SNS and encouraging the parasympathetic nervous system (PNS) "rest and digest" function instead.

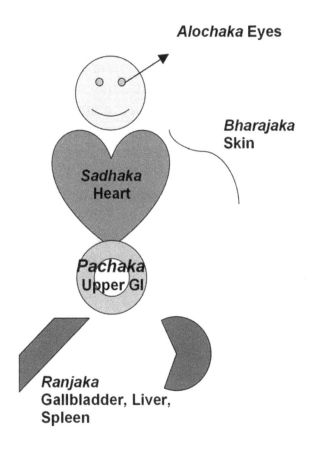

Pitta Dosha Sites

Vata Dosha

The vata dosha is represented by air, with the quality of movement like the wind, and by space consisting of lightness, coolness, and emptiness. The term "ether" is often used instead of space, but because this has the connotation of the anesthetic ether, I prefer the term space. I like to think of this as the space between everything, that also contains everything, including the space between atoms. Unlike the pitta and kapha doshas, vata has no water component, so dryness is a component. Individuals whose dominant dosha is vata tend to be taller or shorter than average, thin with cool, dry skin, and have quick active minds. Hair tends to be kinky or curly; the eyes are small and darting. Intelligence is high with quick understanding, but memory may not be so good. The nervous system, the sense organs, and excretion/elimination, especially by the colon, are important components. Vata is responsible for the movement of energy within our bodies.

When vata is in excess, constipation (from insufficient moisture) and flatulence (from excess space/air) may occur. Anxiety or fear may be present due to too much worrying and inability to stop the mind from fretting. The term "space cadet" can be applied to vata types, who are frequently too much "in their own heads." They are often prone to distractions and impulsive, with a tendency to multitask and to leap ahead of others in their thought process. As a vata type myself, I have the habit of wanting to finish other people's sentences for them, especially if they pause or are slow in speech, as my mind has already formed the words. Waking up in the middle of the night with insomnia due to worrying is a symptom of a stressed vata type. Sometimes the mind is so restless, this type can forget to eat, resulting in difficulty maintaining weight. Vata imbalances tend to arise in the fall and early winter when the weather is typically cool, dry, and breezy.

Dietary treatment for excess vata includes eating warm, moist, heavy foods such as root vegetable stews to provide the missing moisture (water) and heat components. Asana choices that are grounding, such as slower or static postures focusing on the pull of gravity, reduce movement and promote stability. A fast-moving flowing style of asana is often appealing to vata types because they are attracted to movement; however, this fast movement can aggravate a vata imbalance. Vata types do better with a routine schedule and in a warm, humid environment.

Vata has five subdivisions, each of which is named a different *vayu*, which means "wind" or "air." The vata *vayus* describe the directions of the flow of energy or movement in the body. These *vayus* are given more weight and attention in yoga than the subdivisions of kapha and pitta, so more discussion is devoted to them here.

Prana is a Sanskrit term for "life force" or "energy," described in Hindu philosophy as permeating throughout the universe. The word prana also has different uses or connotations in yoga, such as the study of the breath in the word pranayama. In the human body, prana also refers to the movement and energy on which all body functions depend, represented by the five vata *vayus*.

The first of these vata *vayus* is (somewhat confusingly) called the *prana vayu*. The *prana vayu* governs the intake of food and breath, oxygen being our most important immediate source of energy. I think of the *prana vayu* as moving energy into the body. As we inhale, oxygen is provided to the lungs. Oxygen tags on to red blood cells in the capillaries of the lungs and is then distributed via the arterial circulation throughout the body to the cells. This oxygen is required for energy needed in cellular function. Without oxygen, our cells start dying quickly. The breath and oxygen relating to the *prana vayu* can be thought of as the most vital source of life for the body. Focusing on the breath in meditation practice follows the movement of the *prana vayu*.

The *prana vayu* also governs sense perception for input to the brain, the exception being vision, which is more associated with the pitta dosha. Our sensory input from hearing, smell, taste, and the skin produce perceptions in the brain that can trigger memories and thoughts, simplistically speaking. Using both memory and intelligence, these thoughts may or may not produce actions. Sensations can be visualized as starting with stimulation from energy coming from outside the body, such as sound waves, heat, cold, pressure, or the movement of molecules up the nose to the olfactory bulb (smell receptor). This external energy is perceived by the appropriate receptor and the nerves move the information to our spinal cord and brain, producing a thought process, or in some cases a reflex. If movement is appropriate, that command is sent to the muscles, using energy to produce action in the body. So, energy moves from the incoming stimuli to nerves to perception and thoughts, and then possibly to actions in the body. An example of a reflexive movement is touching something hot automatically causes you to withdraw the hand. Another example involving more perception and memory is hearing a favorite tune may cause you to want to get up and dance or sing. These examples illustrate the movement of energy from one form via our senses to another.

Udana vayu represents upward movement responsible for speech, growth, and expression, located mainly in the lungs and throat. U*dana vayu* influences speech quality and childhood growth; humming utilizes this *vayu*. In Kundalini yoga, the movement of prana up the main energy channel of the *sushumna* to the crown chakra would represent *udana vayu*. This concept will be discussed more in Chapter Six.

Samana vayu represents inward movement, such as absorbing and assimilating food from the gut as well as experiences. *Samana vayu* is located in the stomach and small intestine. The movement of digested food molecules across the small intestine wall into the circulation for transportation to the liver can be considered part of *samana vayu*. The venous and lymphatic systems, moving fluid from the body's periphery to our heart, are other examples of this flow of movement from out to in. Assimilating experiences may be another example of *samana vayu*. Most of us have had times in life when we need to "sleep on it" before deciding how we feel about some outside influence or situation. After we have had a chance to absorb and process the experience, we can check back in with our "gut feeling" before making decisions.

Apana vayu is the downward movement of energy for elimination of waste such as stool, urine, and menses. *Apana vayu* is located in the colon, which is the primary site of the vata dosha. Without this important *vayu* function, wastes and toxins are not disposed of in a timely manner and can accumulate in the colon. In the ayurvedic medicine model, lack of proper *apana vayu* function is an important source of disease. Poor digestion, leading to constipation, can cause toxins to build up and even spread and deposit elsewhere in the body, resulting in disease symptoms in other body sites.

Finally, the *Vyana vayu* is the outward movement of energy, such as the heart moving blood through the arterial vessels out to the periphery of the body. As discussed earlier, oxygen from the lungs is absorbed into the red blood cells and then circulated to the body via the arterial system. This outward movement goes from the center of our body to the periphery, including to every cell along the way. Similarly, after the liver transforms our food components into molecules that cells can utilize, these molecules enter the circulation, go to the heart, and then are pumped out to the rest of the body. This energy provided by food is moved outward to feed the cells in the body. The *Vyana vayu* can also be thought of as heat coming from the skin and electromagnetic waves such as EKGs radiating out from the body. The movement of commands from the central nervous system (brain) out to the body via the efferent nerves is also an example of the *vyana vayu*.

The following figure represents the sites of the vata *vayus*. In the chart that follows the figure, I also correlate the subdoshas of vata, pita, and kapha with Western medicine specialties. This chart is meant to link the ayurvedic subdosha concepts, Western medicine specialties, and their corresponding areas of concern. The human mind loves to organize concepts into discrete categories to help us understand how they function. However, in ayurvedic medicine, all these sites and subdivisions are interrelated and not thought of as separate entities.

Vata Vayus Sites

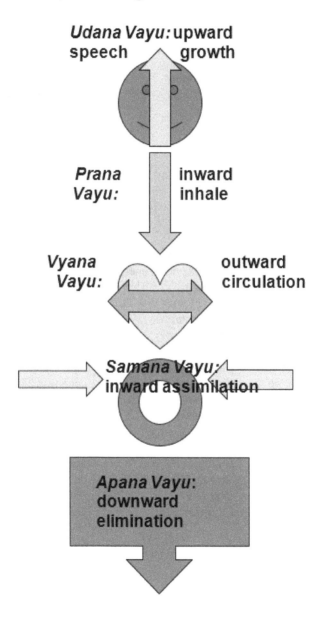

Udana Vayu: upward
speech   growth

*Prana
Vayu:*   inward
            inhale

*Vyana
Vayu:*   outward
            circulation

Samana Vayu:
inward assimilation

Apana Vayu:
downward
elimination

Comparing Subdoshas with Western Medical Specialties

KAPHA	PITTA	VATA VAYUS
Tarpaka: head and cerebrospinal fluid, calmness ENT, neurology, psychology	Alochaka: eyes, vision, and absorbing experiences Ophthalmology and psychology	Prana Vayu: brain and chest, movement for intake of air for oxygen, food, and sensory input to the brain Pulmonology, cardiology, gastroenterology, psychology
Bodhaka: mouth and tongue, taste, and salivation ENT	Sadhaka: heart, emotions Psychology, cardiology	Udana Vayu: throat, upward movement for speech and growth ENT, endocrinology, pediatrics
Avakambhaka: chest, heart, lungs, lubrication, and strength Pulmonary and cardiology	Pachaka: upper gastrointestinal, energy for absorption of food for energy Gastroenterology, endocrinology	Samana Vayu: stomach, small intestine, inward movement as absorption of food, oxygen into tissues Gastroenterology, pulmonology
Kledaka: upper stomach, liquidation of food, acid breakdown Gastroenterology	Ranijaka: liver, spleen, gallbladder, color to stool, blood production Hematology and gastroenterology	Vyana Vayu: cardiovascular, outward movement distribution to tissues via arteries, efferent nerves Cardiology, neurology
Shleshaka: joints, lubrication Orthopedics, rheumatology	Bharajaka: skin, temperature, and moisture Dermatology	Apana Vayu: colon, downward movement, childbirth, evacuation of gut/bladder, menses Gastroenterology and OB/GYN

As discussed above, the three doshas have their subdivisions in the locations within the body that represent different body functions and symptoms when disturbed. In Western medicine, specialists deal virtually exclusively with their area of expertise in certain areas or specific systems of the body. In both ayurvedic and Western medicine, symptoms associated with distinct parts of the body dictate treatment. However, in ayurvedic medicine the patient is treated holistically rather than focusing only on the one area that is presenting with symptoms.

Western medicine often describes staging of disease progression, used for example in conditions such as cancer and heart disease. The various stages represent the severity of the illness, which in turn dictates treatment and prognosis. In ayurvedic medicine, diseases are also thought of as going through stages.[xvii] The initial stage of a disease is thought to be caused by stagnation of toxins in a subdivision of whichever dosha is rising. For example, the *apana vayu* in the colon can be an instigator of the disease process. Undigested food in the colon causes the accumulation of toxins, called *ama*, which can present as constipation, irritable bowel, or diverticulitis. The accumulation of *ama* can overwhelm the bowel, getting into the lymphatics and circulation and spreading toxins to other parts of the body. The duration of the initial stagnation and the extent of the spreading dictates how hard the disease is to treat, just as in the Western model of staging of diseases. A goal of ayurvedic medicine is to treat symptoms early in disease progression or, better yet, to prevent the stagnation from happening in the first place. The accumulation of *ama* gets harder to treat if prolonged or once it has spread. An example of this concept that relates to both ayurvedic and Western medicine is cancer. If caught early and localized, many cancers are curable, whereas metastatic cancer is much harder to treat.

Treatment modalities common to both ayurvedic and Western medicine include dietary and lifestyle recommendations. For example, someone with heartburn and high blood pressure, which can be symptoms of excess pitta, would be advised by both Western and ayurvedic practitioners to avoid spicy foods, caffeine, and alcohol, and to decrease competitive stressors in life. A sedentary person with excess of kapha influence, presenting with weight gain and lethargy, would be encouraged by both types of practitioners to avoid carbohydrates, exercise more, and embrace activity. A vata exacerbation with weight loss and anxiety would be advised more nourishing foods such as warm carbohydrates and a relaxed, structured lifestyle.

Imagery visualization can be beneficial for all three doshas, with a different focus appropriate for each dosha. A vata type may want to imagine someplace warm and moist, such as lying on a sandy tropical beach, to counteract the inherent cold, dry qualities of too much air, movement, and space that characterize an imbalance of vata. A pitta type might envision a high-altitude mountain top, which is cool and dry, to counter the hot, moist qualities of excessive fire and water. And a kapha type could focus on an image of a warm, dry desert sky to offset the inherent moistness, coolness, and heaviness of excessive earth and water. Creating the mental scene by engaging the senses and imagining what you would see, hear, smell, taste, and feel can be very therapeutic.

Ayurveda states that each individual has a constitution, called *prakriti* (or *prakruti*), determined at the time of conception and usually consisting of a mix of all three doshas, with one usually being dominant. For example, a natural constitution may be 60% vata, 30% pitta, and 10% kapha. When we are symptom free, we are in harmony with this predestined ratio. But when we are out of kilter, problems can develop in the balance of the doshas, referred to as *vrikriti*, or our current state of imbalance. Usually, symptoms represent an overactivity of our predominant dosha. Treatments are used to calm down and depress the influence of this rising dosha to return us towards normal.

However, I prefer an alternative approach or attitude towards the doshas. Instead of being "stuck" with our preset dosha ratio, I like to think that we can adjust the ratio depending on our current needs and stages in life. Using ayurvedic tools, we can call up attributes from whichever dosha serves our purpose at that point in time, by incorporating those habits that make it rise. Doing so usually also calms down whichever dosha may be too domineering.

For example, to get the fire and drive to finish this book, I tried to call up my ambitious pitta part to get motivated to write and resume working on it. Energetic spicy foods, active physical practices, and challenging myself mentally helped me pick up the manuscript repeatedly (between long breaks). Each time I started working again, I called on the endurance of my kapha component, being willing to sit and persevere for long hours and several days, inviting calmness and grounding. To encourage these kapha qualities, some overloading on carbs was probably involved too!

My more naturally dominant vata, while creative and the source of many ideas, would get restless and distracted, making it hard to find pitta's drive or kapha's endurance in order to sit down and get the book done. Now, to be honest, eventually my vata would win out; I would have to put the manuscript away for periods of time before starting this process all over again. But the idea of invoking the doshas was helpful to me. I do not think I would have finished the book without using these concepts of the various potentials of pitta and kapha to draw upon, potentials that are not part of my naturally dominant vata traits. This example shows how *svadhyaya* or self-study can help you recognize traits needed during certain times, and then use *tapas* or effort to recruit whatever is helpful in that particular situation.

I like this idea of being able to temporarily adjust the doshas to achieve desired benefit. Doshas tend to fluctuate with the seasons, and we can use ayurvedic tools to counteract the rising dosha if needed. Kapha energy becomes more dominant in the cool, moist spring, pitta rises in the hot, sweaty summer, and vata is exacerbated in the dry, cool fall and early winter. Symptoms associated with a dominance of a dosha are more likely to occur in those respective seasons. Since people are usually mixtures of all three, you can self-treat by reaching for seasonally appropriate diets. For instance, spicy stews are good in the winter when you get cold and dry to counteract vata rising. At the same time, the calories, heat, and warmth of the stews invite pitta's elements of water and fire, providing the heating and moisture qualities that vata lacks.

The three doshas also naturally dominate at various stages of life. Kapha is dominant in childhood, representing growth and structure formation and the beautiful complexions seen in children. Pitta dominates in midlife, firing the drive for careers, the energy for families, and active lifestyles. Then vata dominates in later life as we become older and perhaps less ambitious or driven. The aging body tends to become cooler, dryer, and more brittle, represented by osteoporosis and wrinkled skin. This life progression of aging is natural. However, I like the idea of calling up my pitta or kapha practices to gently counteract my increasing vata qualities as I age.

I do not long for my younger, more energetic years, but to keep in as good of health as possible, I try to keep active and engaged with life. In ayurvedic terms, I embrace practices that produce heat and moisture, rather than the older-age qualities of dryness and coldness representing vata's air and space elements. My tools include food choices (moist and heating), styles of exercise (heating, lubricating, and strengthening), and stimulating mental activities. I remember to allow for times of needed rest provided by earth's grounding quality from my kapha component. But primarily, I embrace energizing activities to encourage pitta's fire and water elements. These practices help keep my dominant vata lubricated and warm.

Ayurvedic medicine is becoming more popular in the West as a form of alternative medicine. Western medicine tends to work well for acute problems, as medications and surgery are often quickly effective. The Western practitioner may begin by prescribing medications, such as those for high blood pressure, to quickly get a condition under control. Ayurvedic medicine may be better for addressing chronic issues, with treatment recommendations that emphasize lifestyle choices, including yoga, meditation, and diet. These treatments may take longer to start working, but eventually may be more effective for treating chronic diseases. Ideally, through the combination of both Western and ayurvedic approaches, the patient's long-term health gradually improves, even to the extent that, under the provider's care, the patient may potentially be weaned off some medications.

When understanding and using the tools for the doshas discussed in this chapter, such as dietary choices, appropriate yoga asanas, imagery, and meditation, long-term health benefits may occur. Incorporating the concepts taught in the *yamas* and *niyamas,* such as *svadhyaya* (self-study), and *ahimsa* (do no harm), may also empower the individual in the quest towards improved health. As in Western medicine, the challenge in ayurvedic medicine can be to get the patient to do the "homework" that involves lifestyle changes. Practicing yoga may incrementally allow the patient to feel the benefits on a physical, mental, and emotional level. This gradual improvement in the quality of life represents positive feedback, which may then encourage the patient to continue practicing yoga and develop lifelong habits that promote health.

Chapter Five: Yoga Concepts

The *Kleshas*

The *kleshas* are "afflictions," or negative patterns of thinking, considered to be obstacles to awareness and to achieving our true potential. The *kleshas* as taught in the *Yoga Sutras* are fundamental causes of pain and suffering. The five *kleshas* are *avidya* (ignorance), *raga* (desire, or attachment to pleasure), *dvesa* (aversion or avoidance)*, abhinivesa* (clinging to our way of life, fear of death), and *asmita* (identifying ourselves with our thinking mind or ego).

Avidya is the ultimate and most influential *klesha*, signifying ignorance of the true spiritual self and misperception of the world. Acting from this *klesha*, we tend to deny our mortality and get caught up in this physical existence, instead of honoring the soul as the true permanent self. Identifying oneself with the materialism of the physical world, outward appearance to others, and thoughts (*asmita*) is habitual for most people. We are defined by jobs, where we live, family background, possessions, and so on. Clinging to material possessions (*raga*) and way of life (*abhinivesa*) results. *Abhinivesa* includes the fear of losing comfortable physical surroundings, fear of losing our self-definition, and more profoundly, the fear of death.

In addition, we identify with the thinking mind, or ego. This "I-am-ness" or maintenance of ego is called *asmita*. We believe our thoughts and feelings are who we really are, when in fact thoughts are even more transient and less substantial than the physical body, which is constantly changing.

The yogic view is that the life force/spirit/soul/*Atman* is the only permanent aspect of our existence, persisting even after biological death. This soul is our true self, not the body, emotions, or thoughts. Recognizing the permanence of the soul while accepting biological mortality can paradoxically free us to pursue a more interesting and fulfilled life.

In past generations, people usually died at home cared for by their loved ones. The modern culture in the United States now tends to shield the actual process of death from the public, with many deaths occurring in hospitals or nursing homes. We may be insulated from death as it is "out of sight, out of mind." If not exposed to death, it is unfamiliar, and more feared. When we do think about it, the thought may be pushed away, and instead the mind turns to cling to physical existence. This fear of loss of ego or loss of definition of self, including loss of mortal life, is called *abvinihesa*.

Instead, it is wise to contemplate death and take assessment of what is profoundly important in life now, rather than waiting for the death bed to sneak up. Trivial worries are just a waste of time and energy. Developing spirituality will open the eyes to the relative unimportance of most of the things that do cause stress. Accepting death as natural may help prioritize, put worries in perspective, and release some stress altogether.

People who are dying value love and relationships, not portfolios or possessions. Love yourself, your family, and your friends now, as the human condition is impermanent. Diminishing fear of death allows the wonderful gift of life to be enjoyed more fully. Identifying with the spiritual self instead of the ego can be wonderfully liberating, in the same sense that it is liberating to sit by the Grand Canyon or under the cosmos at night and realize how insignificant and transient this mortal life is.

Two other *kleshas* are attachment (*raga*) and aversion (*dvesa*), opposite reactions or attitudes to various situations in life. As we grow up and experience life, we are programmed into thinking certain ways about various things, including ourselves. We may have a positive attitude towards something, or conversely a negative attitude. "I hate..." "I love..." "I am good at..." "I am unable to..." are examples of these patterns of thoughts. These learned repetitive thoughts then result in repetitive actions and behavior.

Over time, thoughts and actions that arise from the *kleshas* become repetitive patterns or imprints known as *samskaras*. *Samskaras* have been imposed on us from what others have taught us and from our own experiences. These imprints become habitual thought patterns, like grooves on a vinyl record that play the same tune over and over. Repetition continually reinforces them into more entrenched grooves. Ruminating thoughts are an extreme example of *samskaras*, repetitive thought patterns.

One of the goals of yoga, self-study (*svadhyaya*), is to recognize these patterns and decide which ones may not be serving any good purpose. Then, work can begin on letting go of the negative habitual thought patterns. Releasing the negativity frees open "space" to be replaced with alternative more positive patterns of thought and behavior. Instead of listening to the same old song on rewind mode, to the point that the song becomes stuck in our head, we listen to brand new music and expand our repertoire. New thoughts and input then affect our actions, and we may even learn a new way to dance in life! Recognizing the *samskaras* with their associated attachments (*raga*) or aversions (*dvesa*) expressed in habitual thoughts is the first step. The awareness that arises from paying attention in the present moment to the *samskaras* is the key to both recognizing them and letting them go.

A couple of personal examples from my own life might be helpful here. As a college student, I had no idea what I wanted to do. Fortunately, life connected me with a fellow student who became a lifelong friend. She knew she wanted to be a doctor and started taking me to pre-med meetings with her. As I became interested, the health profession sounded like a steady career with constant demand for services. I liked the idea of helping people, so I decided to pursue it. However, I told myself that I was not smart enough to be a doctor. I am not sure why, but being a physician was not in my self-image, despite always having excellent grades. Perhaps it was the lack of medical role models in my family or acquaintances. I, as an individual, was not defined in that way in my head, so I told myself "I can't be a doctor" and never seriously questioned it.

I decided to become a physician assistant (PA), which was a wonderful life experience, for which I have absolutely no regrets. But it was several years before I developed the confidence to go back to medical school. I certainly loved my life as a PA, but in retrospect something held me back from applying to medical school earlier. I now believe that a limiting thought pattern, or *samskara,* influenced my behavior at age 21, which I eventually saw to be untrue.

Another personal example of overcoming *samskaras* is starting my career later in life as a yoga teacher. The idea of teaching yoga appealed to me, but I believed I was not a good public speaker, probably stemming from an event in third grade.

I had been chosen to portray the nun teaching my class for a PTA skit. My script was crucial to the flow of the play, but I messed up and skipped over the bulk of the script during the live performance. The result felt like a catastrophe to me, and I felt mortified for all the kids who did not get to say their lines. I cried bitterly, though honestly, it probably was of little importance to anyone else involved. However, in my mind I had utterly failed, and I became terrified of speaking in front of a crowd.

For many years, I avoided any public speaking opportunities, such as speech, debate, or plays. However, teaching yoga would involve leading classes verbally and even worse, a group of people looking at me. When I learned of the concepts of *samskaras*, and aversions *(raga),* I reflected on whether I truly was unable to speak in front of an audience. I had never really given myself another chance. I realized that even if I was never good at public speaking, letting go of the idea that I had to be perfect at it was liberating. I had been trying to protect my ego, *asmita*, instead of following my heart's desire *(sankalpa)*. The concept of misidentifying myself with my ego or thoughts was profoundly helpful for me. If my heart was desiring something, why let my ego or definition of myself get in the way?

So, consider letting go of clinging to unhelpful or limiting patterns of thought. Try to stop worrying about massaging the ego or what others think. Acknowledge feeling fear from the possibility of losing the current definition of yourself. Then, after weighing risks, perhaps instead welcome challenges and opportunities to change and evolve. Eventually, even I got over the tongue-tied jitters of a new yoga teacher and have loved sharing my passion with others ever since.

These concepts can be applied to even trivial things in life. Since childhood we have learned to associate liking/clinging or disliking/aversion with objects, experiences, and sensations. For example, perhaps you "hate the cold." You have learned to attach an emotion to an experience, such as hatred being attached to the physical sensation of coldness. The connection is then repeated in your mind over and over, such as "I hate the cold; I hate the cold." Consider the opposite and you may break the negative habitual pattern of thought. Next time you are cold, try feeling the sensation without attaching an emotion to it, like hate, or a thought such as "I hate being cold." Disassociating those habits of thought from the actual experience of direct sensation may be a new way of experiencing the cold for you.

You may want to explore taking this idea further to pursue your goals. Maybe you *can* … fill in the blank. You never know unless you try. It helps to remember the concept of not being attached (*raga*) to the goal itself, but to be content (*santosha*) with the effort (*tapas*) and watch life unfold in new and interesting ways. You may even find that the goal changes as you develop your potential and passions.

To summarize, the *kleshas* teach us that ignorance (*avidya*) of true self is the main obstacle to awareness, as we identify with our thoughts and ego (*asmita*), rather than with our spiritual self. Attachment (*raga*) to concepts of happiness defined by clinging (*abhinivesa*) to this material world result. Aversions (*dvesa*) to things we have told ourselves we do not like or cannot do also come into play. Trying to be aware of the *kleshas* is the first step towards trying to release them. This world is constantly changing, including our aging bodies. Identifying primarily with the spiritual self instead of the body, thoughts, ego, likes, dislikes, possessions, jobs, or titles, may help us age more gracefully and fear death less.

The true self is the spirit, that constant observer. I believe the soul imprints and absorbs this lifetime. I choose to absorb some joy and bliss and release some anxiety. Death is not to be feared (*abhinivesa*), but rather life is to be enjoyed, experienced with wonder and gratitude. Death then becomes a curiosity, an exploration of a mystery, and perhaps even a release or liberation.

"Man often becomes what he believes himself to be. If I keep on saying to myself that I cannot do a certain thing, it is possible that I may end by really becoming incapable of doing it. On the contrary, if I have the belief that I can do it, I shall surely acquire the capacity to do it even if I may not have it at the beginning."

~ Mahatma Gandhi

"Emancipate yourselves from mental slavery, none but ourselves can free our minds!"

~ Bob Marley

The *Koshas* – Sheaths of an Individual

The *koshas* are a way of thinking about individuals as five layers or sheaths (*panchamayakosha*), originally outlined in the *Tiattrirya Upanishad*. The five *koshas* consist of the physical body, the energetic self, the mental self, the intelligence, and finally the bliss layer that veils the spirit or soul. The *koshas* are conceived of as being permeable sheaths that communicate with and percolate through each other, rather than as separate, walled-off, layered compartments. Meditation and self-awareness can help the deeper layers become more accessible to our lived experience.

The outermost layer, called the *annamaya kosha*, consists of the body we can see, touch, feel, and feed. Part of developing self-awareness is becoming embodied, sensing what is happening in the body and how it is connected to the mind. Next is the *pranamaya kosha,* consisting of vital energy, or the life force. This sheath is thought to animate the body, allowing for movement within the body and for life itself. Physical, mental, and metabolic functions are all dependent on *pranamaya kosha*. We can experience the *annamaya* and *pranamaya koshas* as the energetic feeling in the body produced by doing asanas.

The third layer is the *manomaya kosha*, which can be equated with the mind, including thoughts, images, beliefs, and other mental structures. The *manomaya kosha* is the realm of the *samskaras* discussed earlier in this chapter. Transient emotions and moods also reside in this layer. Subtler is the next layer, the *vijnanamaya kosha*, representing intelligence, wisdom, and will. How we choose to act in life is not only a result of transient thoughts, memories, knowledge, and sensations. The wisdom of the *vijnanamaya kosha* allows us to reflect before responding, rather than instinctively reacting to stimuli or thoughts. In Western medicine, the frontal lobe (executive center) of the brain represents this function as it interacts with other parts of the brain. The wise saying of 'count to ten' before reacting gives this layer time to work.

The final, most subtle layer is the *anandamaya kosha*, or "bliss" layer, surrounding and reflecting your *Atman* or spirit. As we go deeper towards this true permanent self, as discussed above in the *kleshas*, bliss becomes the feeling experienced. More frequent visits with meditation and self-awareness result in more frequent moments of bliss, and a more joyful life from experiencing this innermost self.

A metaphor for the koshas is found in the *Bhagavad Gita*, describing a chariot that is being pulled by five horses, their reins, a charioteer, and the passenger. The chariot, horses, reins, charioteer, and passenger represent the body, the senses, the mind, the intelligence, and the soul, respectively. The five horses are the five senses, which if left unchecked can run wild. The reins represent the mind receiving and sending information back and forth between the horses and the charioteer. The charioteer represents intelligence, choosing where to guide the chariot by controlling the mind through the reins, and in turn controlling the senses (horses). The body is the chariot, its direction and action affected by all the above. And, finally, sitting in the chariot, observing it all, is the passenger, the soul or *Atman*, a silent witness. Without the intelligence, the mind and senses are left to their own desires and can run wild and cause havoc to all. But using the intelligence and its willpower, the course is set for the destination desired, as the soul watches and observes all.

The Gross, Subtle, and Causal Bodies

The *Upanishads* and the *Bhagavad Gita* discuss the concepts of the gross, subtle, and causal bodies. These concepts can be considered subgroupings of the *koshas*, progressing from the physical body, to the energetic and thinking levels, then to the spiritual level. The gross body refers to the physical body, represented by the *annamaya kosha*. The subtle body consists of the *pranamaya*, the *manomaya*, and the *vijnanamaya koshas*. The subtle body is felt to be the vehicle of consciousness and ego. Finally, the *anandamaya kosha* is the causal body, the bliss layer veiling the soul or *Atman*.

The tools of yoga may help you access these layers. Keeping the physical and mental body healthy with lifestyle, asana, and pranayama facilitates access to the deeper layers. Asana directly affects the physical body. Progression by using breath (pranayama), mindfulness, and meditation techniques (*pratyahara, dharana*) for the subtle body may then lead to the blissful causal body (*dhyana, samadhi*). Releasing *samskaras* and desires from the gross and subtle layers aide with immersion towards episodes of experiencing this blissful causal layer.

Annamaya	Pranamaya	Manomaya	Vijnanamaya	Anandamaya
Physical body	Energetic body Vitality Breath	Mental body Thoughts	Intelligence Wisdom Will	Bliss Layer
Gross	Subtle	Subtle	Subtle	Causal
Asana	Pranayama	Pratyahara	Dharana	Dhyana to Samadhi

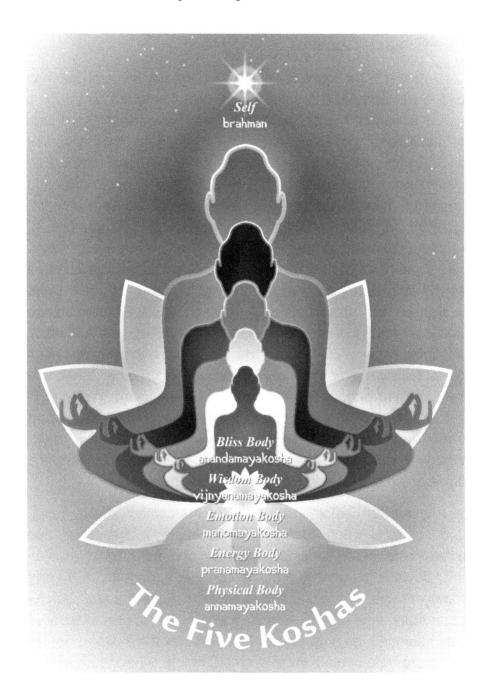

Self
brahman

Bliss Body
anandamayakosha
Wisdom Body
vijnyanamayakosha
Emotion Body
manomayakosha
Energy Body
pranamayakosha
Physical Body
annamayakosha

The Five Koshas

The *Gunas* - Qualities of Nature

Another yoga concept discussed in the *Samkhya* philosophy and the *Bhagavad Gita* important to mention is the *gunas*. The *gunas* of *sattva, tamas*, and *rajas* consist of three different sets of qualities or properties inherent in everything that comprises the universe, including humans. The *gunas* are constantly in flux. *Sattva* is characterized by balance, harmony, goodness, and positivity. *Tamas* has the qualities of being impure, stagnant, ignorant, negative, chaotic, and destructive. The qualities of *rajas* are passion, anger, drive, action, and self-centeredness. All people have each of these tendencies within, and which *guna* comes into dominance is a complex interplay of our outside influences and internal state. How we choose to act reflects the dominant *guna* at that point in time within us. The idea is to enjoy the times of harmony from *sattva,* while understanding that *rajas* gives us energy and drive, and accepting that at times the lethargy and negativity of *tamas* can be dominant. We tend to cycle through the *gunas* depending on how we react to the world around us. Yoga practice can help us achieve a *sattvic* state, though it will most likely be transient, as we later experience times of excess energy (*rajas)* or fatigue (*tamas*).

Ayurvedic medicine also uses the concepts of *sattva, rajas*, and *tamas* to apply to food. For example, rotting foods and excess alcohol are considered *tamasic* and are to be avoided as they deplete our energy. Foods such as peppers and hot spicy foods are *rajasic*, heating and energizing. *Sattvic* foods, such as fresh fruits, vegetables, nuts, and whole grains, are considered well balanced, easy to digest, and good for the system. *Sattvic* foods promote peacefulness and well-being. What we choose to eat affects us physically and mentally.

Recalling the doshas, the *guna* category that a food falls into may aggravate or help an overactive dosha. For example, a rising pitta has excess heat, so a spicey *rajasic* diet would aggravate this and should be avoided. Symptoms of excess kapha are lethargy and coolness, so in that case an activating *rajasic* diet may be beneficial for a period of time, in order to introduce energizing heat from the food. Ideally a *sattvic* diet would be practiced by all three doshas since those foods are the healthiest for our bodies. Please consult an ayurvedic text to see which foods fit into the various categories and are beneficial to specific doshas.

The *Gunas*, Diet, and the Gut

Our nervous system is divided into two branches, the central nervous system (CNS) and the peripheral nervous system. The CNS includes the brain and the spinal cord, and the peripheral nervous system is everything outside the brain and spinal cord. This peripheral nervous system is subdivided into the autonomic nervous system (ANS) and the somatic nervous system. The somatic branch provides for voluntary movement and responses that we have conscious control over. The ANS, on the other hand, works in the background without conscious effort, and controls things like the heart rate, blood pressure, hormones, and the gut.

The ANS is divided into the sympathetic nervous system (SNS), the parasympathetic nervous system (PNS), and the gut's enteric nervous system (ENS). The SNS is referred to as the "fight or flight" system, activating in nature. The PNS is known as the "rest-and-digest" branch, responsible for digestion and assisting with healing and immune function. The peripheral nervous system is also composed of efferent and afferent nerves. Efferent nerves send information from the CNS out to the body, giving commands. Afferent nerves send information such as sensations from the body to the CNS.

We will now turn our attention to the enteric nervous system (ENS) of the gut, part of the autonomic nervous system (ANS). Remembering that the PNS is the "rest and digest" system, it is not surprising that the ENS has a huge interplay with the PNS. The main conduit is via the large, meandering PNS vagus nerve. The vagus starts bilaterally from the brain stem, passing down the neck (pharynx and larynx) and thorax (heart and lungs) to the abdomen (gut). Significant for the mind-body connection, only about 20% of the vagal fibers are composed of efferent fibers (brain to vagus), meaning that approximately 80% of vagus nerve consists of afferent fibers, which send information from the body to the brain.

The vagus nerve is the "major player" nerve connecting the CNS and the gut, sending the brain an immense amount of information, most of which you are never consciously aware. The gut, in this context, includes the stomach, liver, gallbladder, pancreas, intestines, and colon. The gut not only controls digestion and elimination, but it is also our largest endocrine organ, producing important enzymes and hormones. Scientists estimate that about 90% of our serotonin, a mood stabilizer, is produced in the gut. The ENS is also an important part of our immune system. The ENS performs some functions on its own, independent of the CNS input.

Fascinating new research on the ENS regarding anti-inflammatory diets is being done. Distinct types of food interact differently with a variety of gut microbes, which are bacteria that reside in the gut. To put it simply, we all have bacteria in our gut. Some are "good" bacteria providing important benefits, and some are potentially harmful bacteria. Certain kinds of foods feed the beneficial bacteria, which then produce beneficial results in our bodies. Conversely, inflammatory foods feed the "bad" bacteria to trigger production of harmful substances. In terms of the *gunas*, certain foods are beneficial or *sattvic*, and certain foods are inflammatory or *tamasic*. Depending on what foods are ingested, certain types of bacteria may be stimulated to produce various substances that affect the brain, which then affects the mental functioning and the body in specific ways.

If an inflammatory diet is eaten, inflammatory hormones and particles are produced by some of the bacteria. These substances trigger afferent nerve signals via the vagus nerve to the brain. Some hormones and particles that the bacteria produce can also make the gut "leaky" and get into the circulation, traveling up to your brain via the bloodstream. The brain detects this input from the vagus nerve or the particles in the circulation, then gives signals and commands that trigger inflammation in the body.

Chronic inflammation is increasingly thought to be the underlying cause of many medical problems, including heart disease, obesity, type 2 diabetes, arthritis, bowel diseases, and cancer. We discussed how chronic stress can trigger inflammation in Chapter Two. Acute inflammation represents the body's innate immune system response to stressors to protect us from invaders such as bacteria and viruses. Acute inflammation is the "first responder" for tissue injury and is helpful. However, when inflammation becomes chronic, the body continues to believe that it is under attack, and our own cells may become casualties. Research has indicated that inflammation can be triggered by poor food choices, such as highly processed foods, considered to be *tamasic* in ayurvedic medicine, increasing the odds of flaring up illnesses.

Simplistically, if an anti-inflammatory diet is chosen, the "bad" bacteria do not produce these harmful substances, so the brain is not triggered to produce inflammation in the body. An anti-inflammatory *sattvic* diet may affect the sympathetic nervous system (SNS) branch of the ANS by downregulating it, lowering stress hormones. The parasympathetic "rest-and-digest" nervous system is favored with a *sattvic* diet, so your digestion and immune function improves. This beneficial cascade gives the body time to heal and may calm chronic inflammatory diseases such as rheumatoid arthritis, type 2 diabetes, and heart disease.[xviii] You may be less susceptible to illnesses and recuperate quicker if you do get sick.

If you want to learn more about anti-inflammatory diets, I suggest you research this rapidly evolving subject. Sites such as *health.harvard.edu* or *mayoclinic.org* list foods that are beneficial and foods to avoid. As always, check with your healthcare provider before making changes in your diet.

The dietary feedback to the brain by microbes (bacteria) via cytokines, neurotransmitters, and the parasympathetic vagus nerve has a huge interplay on the body and state of health. This new evidence validates the teachings of ayurvedic medicine and the *sattvic* diet that have been passed down for centuries.[xix] Animal studies have shown the importance of the microbiome (the community or types of bacteria active in the gut) to the gut-brain connection. The type of food consumed, interacting with the microbiome, impacts neurotransmitters like melatonin, important for our sleep cycles, and serotonin. Serotonin, which produces a favorable mood in the brain, is mainly produced in the gut and production is favored by foods considered *sattvic*. The anti-inflammatory diet being studied in modern medicine today as an aid for conditions such as irritable bowel and mood disorders is essentially the same *sattvic* diet used in ayurvedic medicine for centuries. Hippocrates himself said, "Let food be thy medicine and medicine be thy food." It is of profound importance to our well-being that we choose our food wisely.

Chapter Six:
The *Chakras* and the *Nadis*

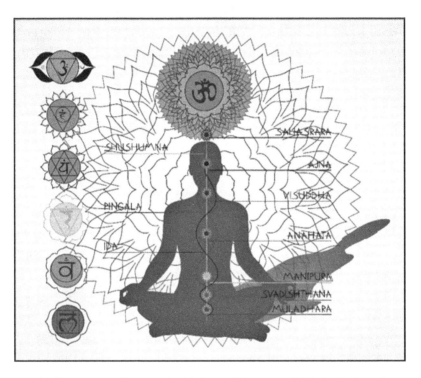

"Matter is Energy ... Energy is Light ... We are all Light Beings"
~ Albert Einstein

The *chakras* and *nadis* can be thought of as a way of organizing the energy flowing in the gross (physical), subtle (energetic, mental, wisdom), and causal (spiritual) selves that were discussed in the last chapter. Mentioned in ancient texts such as the *Vedas* and *Upanishads*, *chakras* are wheels of energy within the body, and *nadis* are the connecting communicating channels. You might visualize the *chakras* as traffic circles with roads (*nadis*) coming in and out. While *chakras* and *nadis* are subtle concepts and cannot be seen, dissected, or imaged radiographically, they do have correlations with anatomy, the ANS, and the neuroendocrine system, which I will address. I like to think of *chakras* and *nadis* as the energy from electrochemical waves that produce nerve impulses flowing in our bodies. For convenience's sake, I will no longer italicize the word chakra.

Yogic texts describe the *sushumna nadi* as the main central channel that runs longitudinally from the crown of the head to the coccyx or pelvic floor and can be correlated with the brain and the cerebral spinal cord. The *sushumna* is the most important energy channel in the body. One of the goals of yoga is to have the prana, or lifeforce energy, flowing freely through the *sushumna* and chakras without obstructions. The *sushumna* connects seven major chakras or energy wheels, from the base or root chakra at the bottom, to the crown chakra at the top of the head. These chakras act like wheels to guide the flow of energy, like old-fashioned water wheels on a stream. The seven chakras should be interacting and flowing smoothly, without blockages (dams) or overdominance (floods) of one chakra. Imagine the water flowing smoothly between all the water wheels on the stream, instead of drenching some areas and depleting others. Examples of causes of blockages are lifestyle habits, belief systems, experiences including trauma, and outside influences.

To the right of the *sushumna* is another longitudinal channel called the *pingala*, representing heat, activation, solar, and masculine qualities, correlating with the sympathetic nervous system (SNS). The *pingala* starts at the root chakra and exits the right nostril. Conversely, the *ida* is a left-sided longitudinal channel representing cooling, lunar, relaxation, and feminine qualities, like the parasympathetic nervous system (PNS) which is responsible for rest, healing, immune function, and digestion. The *ida* also starts at the root chakra but exits the left nostril. These two channels weave around the *sushumna*, then converge at the third-eye chakra, which is the second chakra from the top. The *pingala* and *ida* then separate again and exit out their respective nostrils, just as the flow from your breath exits from the nostrils.

The chakras, the wheels of prana or energy, provide communication between the *sushumna, pingala,* and *ida* where they intersect. Also emitting from the chakras are smaller *nadis* or energy channels, radiating throughout the body. The *nadis* provide for the flow of prana to and from the body. These smaller peripheral *nadis* could be thought of as the electrochemical flow of energy traveling in afferent nerves (going from the body into the spinal cord and the brain) and efferent nerves (going from the brain and spinal cord out to the body). This energy of your nervous system produces sensation, movement, and thought.

Traditionally, each of the lower five chakras has a characteristic motor function, sensory organ, color, sound, and element associated with it. The sounds associated with the chakras are called "seed" syllables. The lowest chakra, the root chakra (in Sanskrit, *muladhara*) represents our basic survival needs such as food, shelter, security, and feelings of safety. It is represented by the color red, the sound "LAM," the sense of smell, the motor function of waste elimination, and the earth element. Asanas or postures using the gravity of the earth for grounding are associated with the root chakra.

I think of the root chakra as being affected by the quality of care one was given as a child by one's parents or caregivers. If you felt physically and emotionally safe, loved, and cared for as a child, this chakra probably has a solid foundation. To keep it healthy, you need to care for yourself in a loving way, so that you feel safe emotionally and your physical needs are being met as best you can, since you are your own adult caregiver.

Next, above the root chakra, is the sacral or pelvic chakra, called *svadhishthana,* the energy of which affects relationships, emotional needs, pleasure, and creativity. It is associated with sexuality, reproductive function, the color orange, the sound "VAM," the sense of taste, and the element of water. Asanas or postures that move the pelvis stimulate this area. Choosing relationships that nurture, rather than those that demean us, maintains self-worth, and helps keep this chakra healthy.

The solar plexus or *manipura* chakra is associated with fire. The energy for digestion and breakdown of food, as well as assimilation of the food by-products into metabolically usable matter, reside here. The stomach, pancreas, upper gastrointestinal tract, liver, and gallbladder are in this area, all contributing to the digestive fire. Located more posteriorly, the kidneys filter our blood and secrete hormones that affect blood pressure. The adrenals, located just above the kidneys, secrete the SNS hormones epinephrine, norepinephrine, and cortisol. The sense of vision is associated with this chakra. This chakra's color is yellow, the sound is "RAM," and its element is fire. The motor function is walking. Twists and strong heating abdominal exercises stimulate this chakra.

Next, we enter the "higher chakras," which influence fewer physical issues and more complex emotional, mental, and higher-consciousness issues. The *anahata*, or heart chakra, is the gateway to these higher chakras. It governs emotions such as love, gratitude, compassion, and devotion. Your intuitive, emotional, sensitive heart is located here, as well as the thymus, which helps with immune function. The heart is cradled by the surrounding lungs and the diaphragm below. Inhalation lowers the diaphragm and expands the lungs, and during exhalation the diaphragm relaxes and moves back up towards the heart. In effect each breath massages the heart. The style of breathing often reflects the present emotional state, examples being staccato type breathing when sobbing, or breath holding when tense. This variety of movement of the lungs and diaphragm with different emotional states massages the heart in diverse ways. Perhaps this can help partially explain why the heart is associated with emotion; the heart can physically sense our emotional state via the type of movement of the diaphragm.

There are so many colloquialisms relating to the heart regarding emotions and health, such as "heartsick," "broken heart," "a big heart," and "my heart leapt for joy." The visual symbol for Valentine's Day is a heart. Meditating on gratitude is a wonderful way to open this chakra, as gratitude is a positive emotion and can help release negativity. The heart chakra is represented by the color green, the sound "YAM," the sensation of touch, the motor function of grasping including hugging, and the element of air. Backbends with chest opening are good for the *anahata* chakra, bringing energy to the chest area by opening the front and sides of the upper rib cage, and encouraging more breath volume and movement there.

I have an interesting anecdote about the heart chakra. A lovely woman who regularly attended my yoga classes was having difficulty staying still for reclining meditation (*savasana*) at the end of class. Given the choice, she usually spent this time sitting up with her eyes open, not looking relaxed. One night she stayed after class and asked for advice. She had previously lost a child and was afraid that she would be overwhelmed by grief during these quiet times if she allowed herself to let go. Her level of grief produced an agitated state that prevented her from experiencing the intended relaxation at the end of class. The next time we met, I gave her a rock quartz stone to hold onto during *savasana*. She was asked to visualize this quartz as representing her love for her child. She cradled the crystal in her palm, at times massaging it with her fingertips and warming it. The physical sensations of warmth and the smoothness from the stone were comforting to her. I suggested if she started to feel overwhelmed by her grief, then she might try focusing on those physical sensations in her hand to help her to stay grounded in the present moment. Having a body focus protected her from the agitated "monkey mind" that magnified her grief during *savasana*. Using this technique, she could still grieve, but was more in control of the process, thereby allowing some healing without being overwhelmed. Eventually she was able to lie down and find relaxation in *savasana*.

Bringing the awareness to a physical sensation, in this case the smooth, warm rose quartz, is an example of the "bottom up" approach to regulating emotion. The mind can be taught to focus on a physical sensation that invites a feeling of safety whenever disturbing thoughts arise, allowing distress to ease. Interestingly, rose quartz is the crystal commonly felt to represent the heart chakra. Like a worry stone, holding a crystal can be calming because bringing awareness to the sense of touch can be soothing. Using a technique like holding a crystal utilizes both the motor function of the heart *chakra* (grasping), and the *chakra's* sensory function of touch, in this case the feeling of the shape, smoothness, and warmth of the stone.

The throat chakra *vishuddha*, in the vocal cords and thyroid gland region, when balanced helps with communication, self-expression, confidence, and creativity. This chakra is represented by the color blue, the sound "HAM," the sense of hearing, the motor function of speech, and the element of space. Range of motion of the neck, tucking and opening the chin, speech, and pranayama techniques including humming stimulate the throat chakra. Self-confidence is an important part of this chakra, especially for public speaking.

In an earlier chapter, if you recall, I shared the fear of public speaking I had developed as a child. When I learned about this chakra, I decided to meditate on it. I used a humming style of breath called "bee breath," tucked my chin, thought of a clear blue sky, and silently repeated the sound "HAM." I invited confidence instead of fear, and with practice my speaking voice did improve. Gradually my SNS physiological reactions of a fast heartbeat, anxious style of breath, muscle shakes, and wavering voice subsided. This was the result of the chakra meditation as well as forming the emotional intention to develop more confidence. Of course, being prepared by knowing the material is a big part of public speaking. But being able to lower the SNS stress response by meditating, reducing fear, and creating calmness gave me more confidence each time I spoke. I also like to silently repeat the sentence "it's not about me, it's about the message" like a mantra. Less focus on myself and how I look (ego), and more focus on what I want to say to the audience helps me to be less self-conscious in front of a crowd, freeing me to concentrate on the material being presented.

The *ajna* chakra, or "third eye," represents perception, intelligence, discrimination, and the merging of the *pingala* and *ida nadis* with the *sushumna nadi*. Here, the duality of masculine/feminine, sympathetic/parasympathetic, and right brain/left brain connections meet. To me, the *ajna* chakra represents the interplay of neural connections and biofeedback between the pituitary and hypothalamus that govern our neuroendocrine axis, the corpus callosum that connects the right and left brain, and complex interactions between brain structures like the amygdala, hippocampus, insula, and frontal lobe. Simply put, the amygdala, hippocampus, and insula process various sensory input and associate the input with long-term memories of emotional states, such as fear, pain, or pleasure. The frontal lobes communicate too and can override an initial impulsive reaction. Working together, these various parts of the brain access learning, memory, and emotional associations, compare present to past circumstances, and then make choices. It is as if the brain can open several files at once and look at the big picture before deciding responses for the present circumstance. Hopefully, astute perception and intelligence allow us to choose our response wisely.

The color violet and the sound "OM" represent the *ajna* chakra. No element, physical sense, or motor function is associated. However, I personally like to think that all the sensory input to the brain represents this chakra's sensation, and the resultant thoughts and decisions represent its motor functions.

The sound "OM" (sometimes written as "AUM) is often chosen for chanting or meditation. It may be chanted as four parts, "AAAH-OOO-MMM," and the silence between the repetitions. The phonetics, the vibrations, and the silence combined add to the meditative experience. A beautiful teaching is that "OM" represents the sound of the universe vibrating.

The final chakra is the *sahasrara,* or crown chakra. Located around the baby's soft spot (anterior fontanelle), it is believed by some to be where the soul enters and leaves the body, and it represents the connection with the divine. I think of it as my energetic connection with the universe or God. No sound, element, sensory, or motor function is associated with this chakra, and the color is purple or white. A possible physical and endocrine correlation may be the pineal gland, which is sensitive to light and responsible for the conscious versus sleeping state, which we will discuss later. Descartes believed that the pineal was where the soul resided.[xx] Meditating on your spiritual self helps you to connect with this chakra.

A goal in yoga is to strive for the chakras to be open and communicating, instead of blocked or stagnant. Asanas, pranayama, meditation, self-study, awareness, and wise choices can all help with that goal. The seed syllable or sound associated with one chakra can be used as a mantra for meditation to evoke that chakra's energy, along with other characteristics of a chakra. For example, to invite positive emotions of the heart, you could visualize green as if you were in nature and/or chant the seed syllable "YAM." A relaxing, restorative mild backbend asana, such as lying back on a bolster, physically opens the heart area and invites fresh energy to this area. Using slow, full breathing to open the chest more, you might invite gratitude into the heart.

Finally, as mentioned in the example earlier, you could hold something you love or find comforting.

Of note is the fact that various sources disagree about the placement of some of the endocrine functions listed in chakras. Chakras are a conceptualization of energy flow, so some variability of interpretation is understandable. For instance, the pineal is often placed in the *ajna* chakra and the pituitary in the *sahasrara* chakra instead of vice-versa. Some place the gonads in the root chakra and the adrenals in the pelvic chakra. The representations in this book are my medically influenced interpretations based on anatomical and physiological body functions, correlated with the functions of the chakras. For example, the pineal produces melatonin which influences our level of consciousness such as alertness versus sleep. When we meditate, our mental state is affected, and we can even enter a dreamlike state similar to melatonin-induced sleep. Meditation and connection to our spiritual self and the divine is a function of *sahasrara*, the crown chakra, so I feel the pineal is better placed here. The adrenal glands produce powerful SNS hormones that physiologically activate the body, correlating more with the heat and fire of the solar plexus chakra, *manipura*. Though they do produce a small amount of sex hormones, this is a minor role of the adrenals compared to the role of releasing adrenalin for activation and cortisol for increasing blood sugar to meet energy needs.

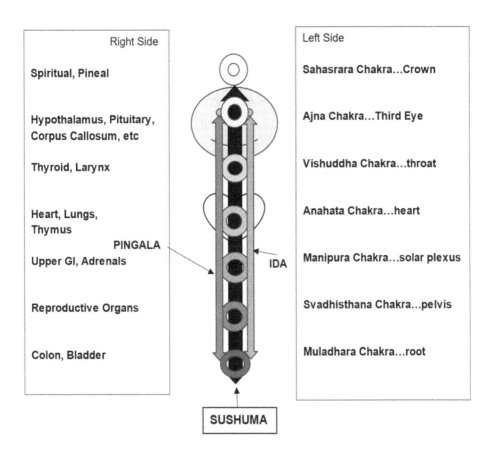

Right Side

Spiritual, Pineal

Hypothalamus, Pituitary, Corpus Callosum, etc

Thyroid, Larynx

Heart, Lungs, Thymus

PINGALA

Upper GI, Adrenals

Reproductive Organs

Colon, Bladder

Left Side

Sahasrara Chakra...Crown

Ajna Chakra...Third Eye

Vishuddha Chakra...throat

Anahata Chakra...heart

Manipura Chakra...solar plexus

IDA

Svadhisthana Chakra...pelvis

Muladhara Chakra...root

SUSHUMA

The Chakras and Nadis

Summary of Chakras

Location	Element	Associate	Sound	Color	Sense & Motor	Endocrine
Sahasrara Crown	None	Spiritually connect with the divine	none	White or violet	Pure consciousness	Pineal
Ajna Third eye	None	Intellect, balance, merging of ida and pingala	OM	Violet or cobalt Blue	Mental clarity	Pituitary, hypothalamus corpus callosum, frontal lobe
Vishuddha Throat	Space ("ether")	Communi-cation, speech, confidence	HAM	Blue	Hearing Speech	Thyroid, parathyroid
Anahata Heart	Air	Emotions	YAM	Green	Touch, grasping	Heart, lungs, thymus
Manipura Solar Plexus	Fire	Energy, drive, ambition	RAM	Yellow	Vision, locomotion	Upper GI, pancreas, liver, adrenals
Svadhish-thana Pelvic	Water	Sexuality, pleasure, relation-ships	VAM	Orange	Taste, reproduction	Gonads
Muladhara Pelvic Floor	Earth	Security, safety, physical needs	LAM	Red	Smell, elimination of waste	Lower GI tract, bladder

Right Brain-Left Brain Correlation with Pingala-Ida

Following is a discussion of right brain/left brain functions and some correlations with the major *nadis*. In general, the right brain controls the left side of the body, and the left brain controls the right side of the body. Therefore, the right-sided, activating *pingala nadi* can be associated with the left-brain hemisphere, and the left-sided, calming *ida nadi* with the right brain hemisphere. The right and left hemispheres of the brain can be thought of as working simultaneously, or in parallel, when trying to decide what to do. They communicate and are physically connected by the corpus callosum, a midline brain structure.

The left brain provides language skills and detailed analytical thinking. Many jobs rely heavily on these skills, for example computer technology. Internal dialogue (thinking in words), analyzing data, and internalized (inward) attention are left-hemispheric dominant functions. The left hemisphere is also responsible for memory that relies on spoken and written experiences. It tends to think of the world in detailed parts. The left brain may also be responsible for self-criticism, rumination, and obsessive thoughts, associated with internal focus and verbal and written memories.

Many of us have a voice frequently running in our head, which may include criticism and judgement of ourselves and others. This voice may represent more of a left-brain function, as mentioned above. If the voice is inducing too much guilt, fear, or anger, we may feel stressed instead of relaxed. As we discussed in the section on the *kleshas*, we can learn to control these self-critical stressful negative patterns of thought (*samskaras*). By releasing negativity and gradually developing new positive patterns of thought and a compassionate internal dialogue, our brains can be rewired via new neural pathways, which is the mechanism of neuroplasticity. As a result, a chronic state of stress and activation of the SNS may be reduced. In simplistic yogic terms, the pingala function of activation may be soothed.

The right brain hemisphere may be associated with the left-sided (calming) feminine *ida nadi*. The right brain is dominant in visual comprehension, external (outward) attention, spatial relationships, and nonverbal communication (body language). Nonverbal visual and spatial memory—such as remembering places, spatial directions, and experiences—resides more in this side.[xxi] Visual memories stored here may include traumatic ones. Trying to disconnect the trigger of similar sights from these disturbing past visual memories may calm an ingrained stress response and reduce suffering.

The right brain function may be more beneficial for guiding appropriate responses to the external stressors of the modern world since it is responsible for outwardly directed attention. This function allows interaction in a complex way with people and technology, helping us to respond in socially acceptable manners. The right brain tends to look at the big picture and think more holistically. Loving-kindness meditation, sending those intentions out to the entire world, may represent a right brain state of mind. Soothing visual imagery as a form of stress relief is another example of right brain function, favoring the *ida nadi* or PNS.

The Caduceus, the Rod of Asclepius, and the Nadis

Most of us are familiar with the Western medical symbol of the caduceus (upper left image following text), which consists of two snakes intertwined around a staff with wings on top. It is interesting how similar some images of the *sushumna*, *ida*, and *pingala* (upper right image) are to images of the snakes and staff in the caduceus symbol used by medical associations. The sushumna correlates with the staff and the two snakes with the ida and pingala intertwining around it. Ironically, the caduceus is historically associated with Mercury, the Greek god of trade and commerce, so is mistakenly used as a medical symbol. The more historically appropriate medical symbol would be the Rod of Asclepius (lower image), who represented healing in ancient Greece. This symbol has only one snake on the staff.

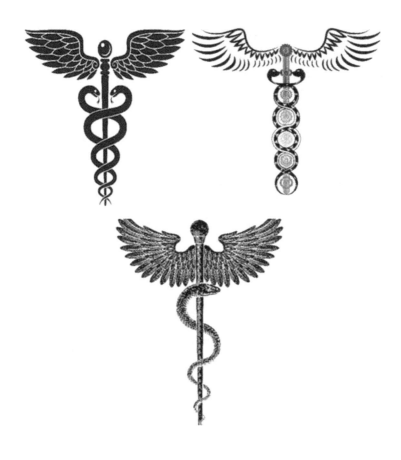

ANS Correlations with the Chakras and Nadis

The correlation of the *pingala/ida* and right-brain/left-brain function was discussed above. It is also fascinating to correlate the chakra system with the autonomic nervous system (ANS), including the sympathetic (SNS) and parasympathetic (PNS) supply to the various areas of the chakras. Abbreviations are used in this section for cervical (C), thoracic (T), lumber (L), and sacral (S) to denote the level of the spine where the nerves enter and exit the spinal cord. The reader may want to refer back to the figure depicting the ANS in Chapter Two.

Of special PNS importance is the tenth cranial nerve, the vagus, which comes from the brain stem and meanders along arteries all the way to the pelvic floor area. Along the way the vagus branches off to the heart, blood vessels, lungs, abdominal organs, and pelvic contents, innervating virtually every organ except the adrenals (which are part of the SNS). Recall the vagus is composed of about 80% afferent nerves, as discussed in the section in the last chapter regarding the *gunas* and the gut. As a review, afferent nerves convey information from the body back up to the central nervous system (the brain and the spinal cord). Afferent nerves send signals such as input and sensations from the environment, or in the case of the vagus nerve, sensations from interoception, what is happening within the body. Efferent nerves conversely run from the brain and spinal cord out to the body, sending motor commands. With only about 20% of the vagus nerve being efferent commands, the afferent vagus nerve has tremendous input and influence on the brain itself.

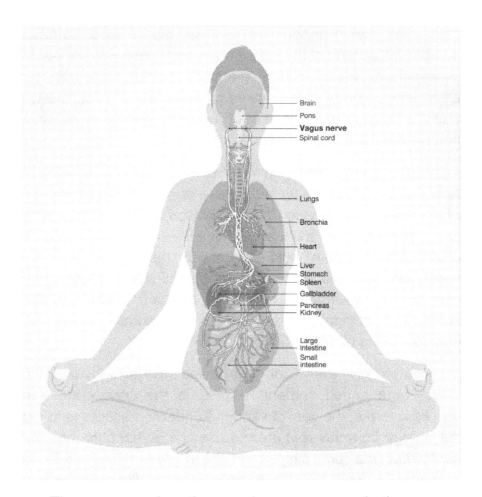

The vagus is the main parasympathetic nerve, intercommunicating along its path with various anatomical nerve plexuses, including some with SNS fibers. Nerve plexuses can be thought of as wads of nervous tissue meeting together and exchanging information. Also included in the PNS, besides the important vagus nerve, are some of the other cranial nerves. These cranial nerves exit directly from the brainstem instead of the spinal cord. Some have PNS function, such as nerves involving the eyes for pupillary constriction and the salivary glands for saliva production to help digest food. Another anatomical location of the PNS is the sacral area, with the pelvic splanchnic nerves arising from the S2-3-4 spinal cord levels. The areas innervated by these nerves correlate with the root chakra and the function of elimination of waste by the gastrointestinal and urinary tracts.

The anatomy of the SNS includes paired ganglia, or wads of nerve tissue, which run up and down along the right and left side of the spine from the neck to the coccyx. Each of these ganglia join with the ones above and below, like two strings of pearls, or chains, providing communication between the ganglia. There are twenty-two right and left pairs of sympathetic ganglia, and at the very bottom an unpaired coccygeal ganglion. There are also some SNS components in some of the cranial nerves, an example being pupillary dilation.

Interestingly, a style of yoga called Kundalini invokes the image of a curled serpent residing in the coccyx area. In simplistic terms, the goal of various Kundalini practices is to get the energy from this root area to rise like a snake through the *sushumna*, *ida*, and pingala via the chakras. Referred to as "Kundalini rising," this life force or energy flows upward to penetrate the crown chakra, merging and uniting the male *pingala* (sympathetic) and female *ida* (parasympathetic) energy channels with the *sushumna*. The possible anatomical correlation of "Kundalini rising" with the electrochemical current of nerve impulses represented by the PNS sacral nerve roots, the vagus nerve, the SNS chains of ganglia, the cranial nerves, and the brain is interesting.

The ANS is a complicated system involving the sympathetic chain and its ganglia, the interwoven nerve plexuses containing both parasympathetic and sympathetic fibers, input to the brain of the wandering vagus nerve, and other cranial nerves' functions. Adding to this complexity is the interplay of the hormonal influence on the brain from various endocrine organs, including the adrenals, and the influence of our food choices on inflammation that we discussed earlier.

The relatively new concept of neuroplasticity involves the ability to reshape the brain by forming new connections between cells and the growth of glial and other support cells. The hippocampus, involved in memory, has shown the ability to grow actual new brain cells. The formation of new synapses (connections between brain cells) provides the opportunity for mental and emotional growth. When I was in medical school, neuroplasticity had not yet been discovered. This ability to reshape the brain validates some of the ancient yoga teachings discussed in the book. In particular, the concept of the *kleshas* and removing negative *samskaras* to promote goals and harmony involves remodeling the brain using neuroplasticity.

Innervations and Hormonal Correlations with Chakras

I discuss in more detail the nerve supply to the various areas corresponding to the chakras, though this material is by no means comprehensive. The following correlations are more anatomically detailed and may not be of interest to some. The basics of the chakras have been covered already, but this next section goes into more depth to correlate neuroanatomy and physiology with the chakras. It is included as some readers (fellow anatomy nerds) may find it interesting and useful as a means to integrate the chakras with the teachings of Western medicine. Others may feel free to skim or skip to the section on Yoga Nidra.

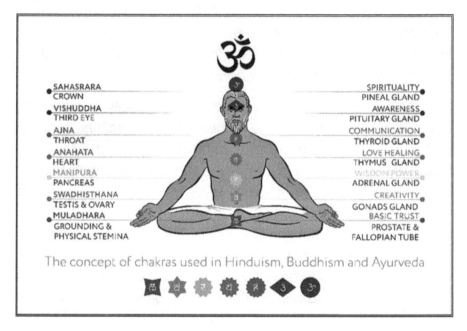

SAHASRARA
CROWN
VISHUDDHA
THIRD EYE
AJNA
THROAT
ANAHATA
HEART
MANIPURA
PANCREAS
SWADHISTHANA
TESTIS & OVARY
MULADHARA
GROUNDING &
PHYSICAL STEMINA

SPIRITUALITY
PINEAL GLAND
AWARENESS
PITUITARY GLAND
COMMUNICATION
THYROID GLAND
LOVE HEALING
THYMUS GLAND
WISDOM POWER
ADRENAL GLAND
CREATIVITY
GONADS GLAND
BASIC TRUST
PROSTATE &
FALLOPIAN TUBE

The concept of chakras used in Hinduism, Buddhism and Ayurveda

The Root Chakra

The root chakra, in the region of the pelvic floor and external genitalia, is innervated by the pudendal nerve, originating at S-3-4, with sensation (afferent), motor (efferent), and some SNS fibers. The rectum has both PNS and SNS fibers. The sexual act involves the sacral PNS nerves for arousal and T12-L2 SNS nerve supply for ejaculation.[xxii] As discussed, the root chakra should provide a feeling of grounding, security, and safety, and is associated with sitting in contact with the earth. The elimination of stool and urine are the main motor functions.

When someone is under extreme threat and unable to escape a dangerous situation, a response is to freeze, along with loss of control of bowel and bladder function. The dorsal vagal nerve—an evolutionally older part of the vagal nerve compared the ventral vagal nerve, which evolved later—is thought to be responsible for this freeze response and the loss of sphincter control. In yogic terms, extreme threat may cause dysfunction in the root charka. For further information, I recommend reading about the fascinating Polyvagal Theory by Dr. Stephen Porges, which discusses the interplay between the dorsal vagal nerve, the SNS, and the (calming) ventral vagus nerve. Irritable bowel and constipation are other examples of stress affecting the root chakra. Conversely, feeling safe and having a well-functioning root chakra make it less likely to have bowel/bladder dysfunction. If caregivers incorporate kindness when potty training children, perhaps healthier bowel and bladder habits may develop.

The Pelvic Chakra

The sacral or pelvic chakra area representing sexuality is in the region of the uterus and pelvic bowl, innervated by the parasympathetic sacral plexus S2-3-4.[xxiii] The hypogastric and ovarian plexus have sympathetic fibers going to and coming from here as well. T 11-L1 also receives afferent nerves from the uterus. That may be why some women get backaches with menses or labor, as the T 11-12 area is in the area of the last two (floating) ribs.

Release and control of our reproductive hormones also depends on the interplay and biofeedback of the ovarian hormones to the hypothalamus and pituitary via the bloodstream. In females, normal monthly cycles occur due to fluctuating ratios of estrogen and progesterone. These ovarian hormones circulate to the brain to influence the secretion of hormones produced by the hypothalamus and pituitary. The brain hormones in turn circulate back to the ovaries to promote regular monthly cycles including menses and ovulation. In yogic terms, biofeedback connects the function of the pelvic chakra with the third-eye chakra. This connection may correlate with how stress, which has a profound effect on the brain, can disrupt normal menstrual cycles. Using stress reduction techniques may help normalize irregular periods and restore fertility.

The Solar Plexus Chakra

The solar chakra's innervation includes the sympathetic celiac and superior mesenteric ganglia from T5-T9, along with the vagus nerve, which combined supply the adrenals, stomach, liver, pancreas, and the intestines.[xxv] This chakra is responsible for transforming food to matter, producing heat and energy. I include the kidneys, which affect blood pressure, and the adrenal glands with this chakra. The adrenals produce epinephrine, norepinephrine, and cortisol. When our SNS kicks in, the first two stress hormones are quickly released into the blood to produce the fight-or-flight response. Cortisol is released more gradually but can last longer. This chakra is represented by the element of fire, which is quite appropriate due to the adrenal release of SNS stress hormones and the powerful digestive hormones from the abdominal organs, such as amylase from the pancreas and acid in the stomach.

The Heart Chakra

Since the heart chakra is associated with touch and grasping, the brachial plexus, which supplies our sensation-rich hands and the motor function to the arms, is an appropriate correlation. The brachial plexus, a complex of nerves, crosses under the clavicles, in front of the upper ribs, on the way back and forth from the arms to the lower cervical and upper thoracic nerve roots, in close approximation to the heart chakra. The emotional act of hugging someone utilizes both the sensory and motor function of the brachial plexus.

The heart and lungs are intimately connected with the ANS. In an instant you can be stimulated by some stressor to activate the SNS. The heart has thoracic sympathetic chain ganglia input from upper thoracic area[xxvi], which along with the adrenal hormones work to increase your heart rate, the volume of blood pumped, and the blood pressure. Blood is shunted from the gut to the muscles, and your style of breath changes to provide for oxygenation of the muscles. Blood sugar (glucose) is released by the liver into the blood for energy. Bronchodilation, opening of the airways, occurs via SNS norepinephrine release, allowing for more air and oxygen exchange.[xxvii]

Conversely, the PNS vagus nerve acts via the cardiac plexus by slowing the heart and breath rates and lowering the blood pressure. The lungs are influenced by the vagus nerve to produce bronchoconstriction and breath rate slows. Blood is shunted back to the organs and gut for digestive processes.

Your emotional state is reflected by these responses. You can feel calm and relaxed (PNS) or alert and vigilant (SNS) depending on which side is dominating at that time. When functioning optimally, the two systems coordinate to create the appropriate level of nervous system arousal to meet whatever happens to be occurring. Since our range of physiological states, including calmness versus agitation, are dramatically affected by the ANS effects on the heart and lungs, it is appropriate that the heart chakra is associated with our emotional state.

The phrenic nerve supplies the diaphragm, the main respiratory muscle, which works with the brainstem to control respiration. Coming from C 3-5,[xxix] with connections with the cervical and brachial plexus, the phrenic nerve supplies motor efferent commands to the diaphragm causing contraction, producing inhalation. The phrenic nerve also receives sensory components from the central tendon of the diaphragm, the mediastinum, and pericardium.

As mentioned, usually breathing is controlled by the ANS, yet we can impose voluntary control of the breath, as in pranayama. Diaphragmatic control is integral to the quality of speech, which represents the throat chakra, making it interesting that the phrenic nerve originates from that area of the neck but travels down to the diaphragm. Confident speaking reflects the ability to project our voice via proper control of the diaphragm, and also is a sign of a well-functioning throat chakra.

An interesting study showed the *right* phrenic nerve has a catecholaminergic (sympathetic) branch below the diaphragm in the abdomen that communicates with the celiac ganglion. The celiac ganglion, residing in an area behind the stomach, serves as an important nerve conduit for the peripheral autonomic nervous system in the abdomen. This SNS branch of the right phrenic nerve communicates with and interacts with the celiac ganglion. On the other hand, in this study, there were no sympathetic fibers noted in the *left* phrenic nerve below the diaphragm.[xxxi] I think this study is an interesting anatomical correlation with the right-sided activating pingala (SNS) and the left-sided cooling ida (PNS).

The thymus gland, located behind the sternum and in front of the heart, is important for immune function, especially T-cell lymphocytes, and some hormone production. The thymus is larger and more active in children and teenagers. Interestingly, it shrinks in size and function with aging. Certain infections, such as HIV, have also been associated with shrinkage of the thymus. Environmental stressors can cause decreased functioning of this gland as well. Perhaps calming parasympathetic yoga practices could help counteract the effect that aging and stress have on the shrinkage of the thymus gland and prolong its immune function benefits.

The Throat Chakra

The throat chakra has ANS input from the SNS cervical chain ganglia, PNS ganglia, and vagus nerve innervation to the larynx (voice box) via the recurrent laryngeal nerve. The phrenic nerve also comes from C 3-5 and travels down to supply the diaphragm, as already mentioned. While the diaphragm helps with projection of the voice, speech itself is a function of the larynx.

Too much SNS stimulation can make you "tongue tied," causing the voice box to feel tight and a dry mouth. As anyone who has experienced fear of public speaking knows, it can feel hard to swallow, as if you have a lump in your throat. Conversely, being prepared and confident in what you have to say promotes relaxation and the parasympathetic mode, downplaying this uncomfortable SNS effect.

The thyroid gland resides in the neck and is responsible for regulating the body's metabolism. Overactivity of this gland increases the metabolism, with symptoms such as anxiety, hyperactivity, weight loss, fast heart rate, and trembling. Low thyroid function produces the opposite symptoms. Just as we want to be able to balance our ANS, we also want our thyroid function to be "not too hot, not too cold, but just right."

The Third-Eye Chakra

The third eye chakra is the commander of brain-body functions, represented hormonally by the hypothalamus and pituitary and their neuroendocrine control. Biofeedback of hormones from various organs, such as the thyroid and ovary, via the circulation to the brain provides fine tuning of our endocrine system. The ANS acts on the brain and vice-versa. We have already discussed how our diet can affect the brain to trigger or calm an inflammatory response in the body.

The interpretation of the sensory input within the brain itself also factors in how the brain perceives a stimulus and decides to respond. Areas of the brain that store memory and emotions (the amygdala and hippocampus), along with right-brain/left-brain functions and the connecting corpus callosum, all interact with the incoming stimulation to communicate with the prefrontal cortex. Given enough time, the prefrontal cortex then assesses the situation and decides what to do, allowing for a thoughtful response rather than an impulsive reaction.

For example, to a veteran who has served in a war, a loud noise could sound like gunfire or a bomb and feel like a current active threat. The stimulus of the loud noise is processed in memory sections of the brain as a danger and may trigger an SNS response, as well as emotions such as fear or anger. But if the veteran is able to pause and allow time for the prefrontal cortex to override the initial impulsive reaction, the SNS "fight or flight" response may be dampened or prevented. By allowing the mind to determine that the stimulus is not threatening, but instead is the sound of a door slamming or a book falling, the prefrontal cortex can choose an appropriate response instead of fear or anger. By reprogramming the interpretation of the sensory input, eventually the sound itself becomes non-threatening. This recircuiting of the brain is an example of neuroplasticity, the brain's ability to change itself. In yoga language, the third-eye is allowed to perceive things clearly and use its intelligence to choose wisely.

"Between stimulus and response there is a space. In that space is our power to choose our response. In our response lies our growth and our freedom."

~ Viktor E. Frankl

The Crown Chakra

The crown chakra represents spirituality and enlightenment. The mysterious pineal gland is located towards the top of the brain. As mentioned, the pineal gland secretes melatonin and is associated with sleep and wakefulness cycles. These circadian rhythms, with changing states of consciousness, are represented by different brain wave patterns throughout the day and night reflected by electroencephalograms, or EEGs. These various levels of consciousness, ranging from wide awake and alert to deep sleep, show different EEG patterns. A discussion follows which includes some studies on meditative states and EEGs. Newer studies are being done using the technology of PET scans, showing pictures of brain activity during different mental states. It will be interesting to see the results of PET scan studies using yoga techniques and how the brain is affected while using specific techniques, as well as long-term remodeling of the brain in yoga practitioners due to neuroplasticity.

EEGs, State of Consciousness, and Meditation

Brains waves as measured by EEGs are electrical fluctuations representing brain activity. These wave patterns are different depending on whether we are wide awake, relaxed, drowsy, falling asleep, or in the various stages of sleep (dreaming, light sleep, deep sleep). Patterns of wavelength frequencies and amplitudes correlate with these various stages of consciousness. There are five major types of EEG waves: beta, alpha, gamma, theta, and delta.

Beta waves are usually present while we are alert, awake, in states of expectation, and fully conscious. They tend to occur when the eyes are open and are active in the frontal and sensory-motor cortex.[xxxii] Beta waves are associated with cognitive function and decision making.

Gamma waves, the fastest wave frequency with the lowest amplitude, and are associated with focused states, such as mindfulness and reaching for an elusive long-term memory.[xxxiii] Gamma waves also briefly fire diffusely in the brain when you have an "aha" moment, such as when you find a solution for a puzzle or remember a word. The brain registers these experiences as pleasant moments, like a self-reward.

Meditating on compassion has been shown to increase gamma waves. One study showed that long-term Buddhist practitioners of loving-kindness and compassion meditation demonstrated increases in gamma waves even at baseline, before starting meditation sessions.[xxxiv] The gamma wave prevalence was also shown to be significantly higher during meditation in these experienced meditators than in the controls. Since the gamma waves were higher in the long-term meditators even while not meditating, this infers that their compassionate mindfulness had become an enduring trait, rather than a transient state happening only during meditation.[xxxv] Practicing compassion and loving-kindness increased their baseline gamma waves, probably via neuroplasticity. This interior trait of compassion and kindness is called the *"dmigs med snying rje"* state of mind by the Tibetans, in which benevolence and compassion pervade the mind as a way of being. Many positive effects have been associated with gamma waves, including increased intelligence, positivity, memory and, of course, compassion.

Alpha waves are associated with a relaxed state that is a bridge between alertness and drowsiness. In adults, this wave frequency is the most dominant pattern. Alpha waves may be seen best on EEGs when the person's eyes are closed while trying to access factual memory. Next time you try to recall something, notice if you closed your eyes while doing so, as it may help you retrieve that elusive fact. Creativity and calmness[xxxvi] are associated with alpha waves.

Theta brain waves occur with drowsiness, REM (rapid eye movement) sleep, dreaming (which usually occurs during periods of REM), daydreams, and some states of meditation. Theta waves happen in a semi-hypnotic state when we are in touch with the subconscious. Theta waves may represent the silent voice within you, such as intuition, insight, and creativity.[xxxvii] This fact may be a good reason to keep a dream journal.

Deeper still towards unconsciousness is the delta wave state, which is the slowest wave pattern, present in deep restorative sleep with minimal consciousness, and in young children. The frontal brain area is associated with delta waves during deep sleep, as if we are solving our problems while nearly unconscious.

Yoga Nidra

The term yoga nidra has been mentioned as early as the *Upanishads*,[xxxviii] referred to as a meditative state of samadhi (bliss). In the 1940's and 1950's, a young man named Swami Satyananda was living at the Bihar School of Yoga in India. He guarded a nearby children's school at night, typically sleeping from 3 am to 6 am. While he was asleep, the children would awaken early each morning and recite their mantras. Later, Swami Satyananda was amazed to discover that he was familiar with these mantras, even though he had never been awake when he had heard them. He became extremely interested in the sleep state and decided to study the practice of yoga nidra, or "yogic sleep," eventually developing his own technique. He borrowed from the Tantra practice of Nyasa Kriya, in which every body part is consecrated while chanting mantras. To simplify the practice and make it more accessible to others, he developed a system now taught throughout the world, during which the teacher verbally guides the practice, instead of the participants chanting. This practice includes the initial preparation of the laying supine in savasana, making an intention or heart's desire (*sankalpa*), rotation of consciousness, awareness of breath, noticing opposite feelings and sensations, and visualization of images. After a period of silence, the participants are asked to recall the *sankalpa* before ending the practice.[xxxix] This technique induces a deep body-mind relaxation with the goal of increasing self-awareness.

There are different variations of yoga nidra practiced today. The technique I describe and use follows the basic outline of Swami Satyananda's teachings. Yoga nidra is usually initiated with the practitioner getting into a comfortable supine position, then being guided verbally by the instructor. At the beginning of the practice, one is asked to choose an intention, a resolution, or a heart's desire (*sankalpa*) and to visualize this as already being true. Cues are given to relax the body and calming breath techniques may be used, such as belly breathing or spinal breath. Usually, the participant's awareness is rotated through different body parts guided by the instructor. The script may then include other imagery cues, such as imagining opposites like heaviness and lightness, then releasing both. Visual imagery may be added, using scenes from nature, before finally a prolonged time of stillness and silence are experienced. The participant usually reaches a relaxed state somewhere between wakefulness and deep sleep. One may feel a loss of the sense of time, as if in a deep sleep, yet still be aware of surroundings. After the period of stillness and silence, the participant is gently guided out of the dream-like state. At the end of the practice, the instructor may ask the participant to recall and meditate upon their heart's desire or intention.

Studies have shown that yoga nidra is associated with brain wave patterns of alpha frequency, the bridge between wakefulness and sleep. Gaining experience in yoga nidra showed an increase in these alpha waves in participants.[xl] Practiced meditators also showed theta waves during yoga nidra alongside the alpha waves, and even the delta waves of a deep sleep. A sense of a relaxed state is reflected in these EEG patterns, demonstrating the interplay of yoga nidra's effect on the conscious and subconscious states of mind.

Dopamine, a brain hormone associated with motivation and wellbeing, was shown to increase during meditation in yoga nidra.[xli] Parkinson's patients are characterized by dopamine deficiency, and it would be interesting to see if they would benefit from this practice. The yoga nidra experience can be wonderfully restful and refreshing, like a power nap, and afterwards people often report feeling like they have been asleep for several hours. Sleep states are known to be associated with healing and improved immune function.

Yoga nidra can allow for insights in self-study. Setting your *sankalpa* can be challenging. The first time I participated in a yoga nidra, I had no idea what my heart's desire was. I decided my *sankalpa* would be to find my heart's desire. Visualizing your *sankalpa* as if it were already true can help you release negative patterns of thought (*samskaras*) that no longer serve you well, opening your true potential to reach your heart's desire. Visualizing the sensation of opposites, such as hot-cold or happy-sad, mimics the extremes of normal life experiences and demonstrates that change and impermanence are part of being human. All these benefits stemming from the practice of yoga nidra may contribute to the health of the body, mind, and spirit.

Chapter Seven:
Asana

"The study of asana is not about mastering posture. It's about using posture to understand and transform yourself."

~ B.K.S Iyengar

Asanas, or postures, may be categorized into anatomical positions of the spine: forward folds (spinal flexion), backbends (spinal extension), side bends (lateral flexion of the spine), twists (spinal rotation), elongation, and neutral spine. The asanas are accompanied by various positions of the pelvis and extremities. We can also categorize asana by body position in space, such as standing, balancing, kneeling, sitting, prone (belly down), supine (belly up), side-lying, and inversions. Asanas have unique benefits that may be used to help specific physical issues as well as more holistic benefits. However, yoga asanas are not like cookbooks with recipes for curing specific illnesses. Rather, the postures are like a toolbox, using a variety of asanas to find whatever helps improve an individual's sense of wellbeing.

Styles of yoga range from highly active gymnastic and power styles such as ashtanga, which can involve jumping, handstands, and arm balances, to more relaxed styles such as Yin and restorative yoga, which may use props and bolsters to support the body in various positions for several minutes of relaxation. Care should be taken in choosing the type of class appropriate for the person's needs and present capabilities. A good instructor, and perhaps individual sessions, assist in safely guiding towards proper alignment of the body during asana practice. Postures may be chosen that are appropriate for an individual's strength, flexibility, and balance, with modifications used as needed.

Yoga therapy, an emerging profession, is designed to help individuals strive for an optimal state of wellbeing by addressing the client's physical, mental, and emotional needs. Asana, the breath (pranayama), meditation, imagery, and introducing yogic concepts are some of the tools used. When I first signed up for my yoga therapy training course, I was expecting protocols of asanas for various ailments such as low-back pain, high blood pressure, and depression. Certain categories of techniques do tend to help certain issues, such as forward folds tend to lower blood pressure. However, finding which asanas are therapeutic for an individual usually is a trial-and-error process, dependent on how the client responds. Different bodies and personalities respond beneficially to one asana, while others may not.

For a yoga therapist, getting feedback from the client is important. The client is encouraged to tune-in to how they are feeling before, during, and after each posture and session. Interoception, the awareness of the sensations coming from within the body, is encouraged for feedback. Interoception examples include the awareness of pain or pleasurable sensations, feelings of stretching versus compression, the position of the body in space, pressure points in contact with the earth, and how the breath reflects ease versus effort. The inward awareness of the body's response to asanas is important for dealing safely with musculoskeletal and other health issues, honoring *ahimsa,* or non-harming.

It is also important for the yoga therapist to assess the emotional and mental effects of yoga practices on clients. What brings release, calmness, and contentment? Or, if the client is feeling lethargic, what brings energy and a more positive outlook? Noticing the feel of the physical body along with the mental effects encourages awareness of the mind-body connection.

A few years ago, I attended a workshop at Duke entitled "Integrative Yoga for Seniors Professional Training." A phrase the instructors used was "gentle is the new advanced." This phrase stuck with me. Yoga asana is not necessarily about mastering the more difficult moves like arm balances or splits. A personal phrase I use for teaching is to suggest releasing the "no pain, no gain" attitude, and instead invite "nurture, not torture." Asana is meant to be an exploration of self, not a competition for the ego.

Forward folds

Forward folds, also called forward bends, imply flexion at the hip and/or spine and are usually relaxing, favoring PNS activation. In general, these types of poses will help reduce anxiety or fatigue. They also stretch the back of the body, including the hamstrings and the back muscles. If done incorrectly, however, forward folds can strain these areas. People are often so interested in gaining flexibility of the hamstrings that they sacrifice the health of the low back. For example, while doing a standing forward fold, one may try to keep the knees straight to stretch the hamstrings while straining forward to touch the toes. If the hamstrings are tight, the pelvis is tilted posteriorly and the low back flexes and rounds. The fronts of the vertebrae are then compressed, potentially aggravating low back problems prevalent in our aging baby-boomer society. If someone has osteoporosis of the spine, sacroiliac issues, or disc problems, flexion of the spine causing compression of the anterior spinal column may be an issue, and modifications should be considered. The spinal flexors including the rectus abdominus may be worked in other positions during which the spine is unloaded, such as properly executed floor exercises to tone the core.

Hip impingement, or femoral-acetabular impingement, may cause damage to the cartilage in the anterior hip joint and can present as pain in the groin region. Hip impingement is related to the individual's shape of the ball and socket joint. Extremes of hip flexion and deep squats may aggravate this condition and should be avoided by those affected. Repetitively overstretching the front of the hip joint while placing the hip joint in extreme extension may also cause problems. The muscles of the hip and back may be strengthened and stretched while avoiding excessive acute hip flexion or extension, to help reduce wear and damage to the cartilage in the front of the joint.

In general, a safe technique to enter a standing forward fold is to flex at the hip joint while also letting the knees bend and the pelvis move posteriorly. The knee flexion allows less extreme hip flexion, and instead of rounding the lumbar spine, the low back stays in neutral and follows the hinging pelvis. As the knees bend, the bottom is sent back into a squat position on the way to the forward fold, releasing tension on the pelvis and lumbar spine, as in the second and third figure below. The normal lumbar lordotic (low back) curve should be maintained, and the spine follows the forward tilt of the pelvis, instead of rounding or flexing. Keeping the hands on the thighs unloads and protects the back.

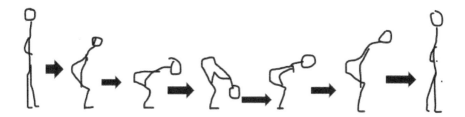

Dropping the bottom back into a squat position on the way back and forth from standing upright to a full forward fold feels like a rocking chair movement. The squat allows the upper body and head weight to stay closer to your center of gravity, protecting the spine and sacroiliac joint. The spine maintains its length until the weight of the head is below the spine. Then, as the head drops, the bottom lifts, and the knees may partially straighten, as in the middle figure above. Once down, the weight of the head can work like traction with the pull of gravity to decompress the vertebrae and discs. Coming back up from the forward fold position (figure five in sequence), drop into a squat (chair pose) as you lift the head to keep a neutral spine. Then assisting with the hands on the thighs, tilt the pelvis back up as the spine follows and the head lifts to an upright position (last two figures).

This technique produces less compression of the anterior vertebrae. Young people with healthy spines and strong bones may be safe with curving or flexing the spine with the weight of the head and upper body on it. I often hear the cue "round down vertebrae by vertebrae." But older adults may have softer bones due to osteoporosis or osteopenia, putting them at increased risk of compression fractures of the vertebrae. Disc disease may also be aggravated by rounding the back, so I am not a fan of the rounding up or down technique for my older population of clients.

Transitions to postures are just as important as the postures themselves. In addition to the rounded back style, I often see another common transition to a forward fold, the cantilever technique. The weight of the head and torso hinge forward, flexing at the hip with a straight spine, but keeping the knees straight. This cantilevering technique places strain on the sacroiliac and lumbar spine, especially if the arms are reaching overhead, which places even more weight away from the body's center of gravity.

Try the gentler rocking chair style yourself while doing forward folds and getting in and out of chairs. When coming up from a chair, place your hands on your thighs and straddle the legs so the torso has room to hinge forward. Gradually the whole hamstring/lumbar fascial connections may loosen so that a full forward fold with straight knees may be possible without causing lumbar flexion or strain. Never force the asana; embrace the shape that you are in.

One of my mantras in class is, "The back is more important than your hamstrings." I also find people may not perform seated forward folds in a safe manner. When sitting on the floor, tightness in the hamstrings or gluteal muscles can "grip" the pelvis, restricting its ability to anteriorly tilt. Instead, the low back flexes and rounds as people reach towards the toes, placing strain on the discs and anterior vertebrae. To counteract this, try sitting on an elevated prop to give more mobility to the pelvis. Keeping the knees bent and the thighs straddled also allow the pelvis and torso to tilt forward, while keeping the spine in neutral.

For someone new to yoga, inflexible, or who may have disc issues or osteoporosis, it may be judicious to introduce forward folds in body positions other than sitting. Sitting on the floor while rounding forward (flexing the spine) puts increased load, measured as pounds per square inch, on the discs and vertebrae. This load increases even more if the back rounds while pulling on a strap looped around the foot. Other body positions with decreased spinal loads can be used to stretch the back muscles and strengthen the abdominal muscles, such as lying on the side, prone, or supine while bringing knees to chest into a fetal position. Hamstrings can be stretched while lying on the back with one leg in the air or placing the legs up the wall, producing less stress on the discs and vertebrae. Modifications can be chosen to fit the client's needs while still achieving desired benefits in a safer manner.

As mentioned above, most forward folds are relaxing and favor the PNS. They tend to lower SNS activities, so may be helpful in patients with conditions associated with excess SNS activity, such as hypertension, anxiety, irritable bowel, and insomnia. For example, child's pose, a prone position with the torso lying on the thighs and bent knees and the weight of the head supported, is a restful pose, as long as the client is comfortable. Sometimes a block under the sitting bones and forehead and a small, rolled towel under the front of the ankles or behind the knees makes this position more accessible to certain body types. When using child's pose as a resting position, I often cue the clients to notice the belly breath, relax the jaw, and guide them verbally through the kosha layers to notice the effect of the posture.

Backbends

Backbends are energizing and favor the SNS. They are great for opening the chest to counter the poor posture of hunched rounded shoulders. Care should be taken not to hyperextend the lower lumbar spine while excessively anteriorly tilting the pelvis, which could compress the posterior aspect of the lowest lumbar vertebrae (the facet joints) and the sacroiliac joint. Engaging strong core and abdominal muscles helps protect this area.

My backbend cues are to first engage the abdominal and gluteal muscles isometrically while keeping the pelvis in a neutral position. Neutral position implies a normal lordotic curve, neither a flat back (posterior pelvic tilt) nor excessive arching of the low back (anterior pelvic tilt). I sometimes use the analogy that you do not want to be the flat-backed cowboy, or the sway-backed horse. Once the spine and pelvis are in neutral, the actual backbend starts when we elongate the upper spine while lifting the chest and rolling the shoulder blades back and down (retracting and lowering the scapulae). Backward extension of the upper lumbar and thoracic spine (reversing the kyphotic curve) results in the "opening" of the chest. Back extension can aggravate spinal stenosis, which is a narrowing of the spinal canal, so it is best to avoid backbends when this condition is present.

Since backbends are invigorating, they may be a tool for yoga therapists to use when working with issues of depression and lethargy. Including backbends may be good for people with predominantly kapha dosha issues, as these people may need to be energized. Physically building strength and confidence, backbends are also considered heart openers and may invite a surge of emotions. In some clients with trauma history, care should be taken as this emotional release may feel overwhelming. Mental health care training is advisable if dealing with this population in order for trauma issues to be handled with in a properly prepared manner.

Sometimes I demonstrate a standing position with a nice open chest and a tall spine, then alternatively demonstrate standing with a sunken chest and the spine and shoulders rounded forward. Then I ask the class, which person would you rather talk to at a party? The posture can show how a person is feeling mentally and emotionally. The inside feelings are reflected on the outside body.

Just as your physical posture reflects how you are feeling, or your mental/emotional state, the opposite is true, too. Your physical posture can affect how you feel mentally. A tall, confident posture sends different signals to your brain than a sunken, slouched one. The effect of proper posture can be a more positive affect, or outlook! Good posture itself can make you feel better both physically and mentally. Another of my personal mantras, "Lead with an open heart," applies to both my physical posture and my attitude towards the world.

Inversions

Inversions reverse the pull of gravity and may be helpful for the flow of fluid in your connective tissue, cerebral spinal fluid, lymphatics, venous system, and intra-abdominal contents. For example, the lymphatics and veins in the legs are below the heart when standing up. As the venous blood and lymphatic fluid need to flow back to the heart, this flow must work against gravity when standing. Reversing the pull of gravity by lying supine and putting the legs up (legs-up-the-wall) can allow these fluids to make their way back to the heart while using gravity as an assist. The valves in the veins that prevent backflow are allowed to open and rest, helpful with varicose veins and fluid retention. However, if someone has congestive heart failure, this position may overload the heart and should be avoided

Inversions can be either relaxing or energizing, depending on the asana. For example, legs-up-the-wall tends to be relaxing and has a forward fold component as discussed above. An invigorating inversion would be a handstand, which involves balance, a backbend, and a component of fear of falling.

Looking at the world upside down may change your psychological perspective about your surroundings and yourself. The first time you do a supported forearm stand, which is a headstand with elbows and forearms supporting the body weight, a feeling of exhilaration occurs, like riding a rollercoaster. The "wow" feeling persists even when you come out of it. You were doing something brand new, seeing and even feeling the world upside down, which is the opposite perspective from your normal upright view. If you are new to the experience, it helps you to realize your potential. This different point of view can be extrapolated to consider unusual ways of looking at life and challenging your ideas of your own limitations.

Incidentally, I am not a fan of doing a headstand without forearm support. The cervical vertebrae are rather delicate to be supporting all that body weight in the tripod variation. With a forearm stand, the arms and shoulder girdle should take most of the body weight, barely allowing the head to touch the floor, depending on the length of your arms.

Supported, resting inversions, such as the popular legs-up-the-wall pose, usually feel good to the back, so may be useful in patients with lumbar strain, disc disease, and osteoarthritis of the spine to ease symptoms. Down dog is another common asana, an inverted "v" shape of the body with the pelvis lifted and the hands and feet on the floor. If done correctly, this position allows for elongation of the spine with the weight of the head acting like traction, and may improve some back pain symptoms, as well as strengthening the shoulder girdle.

Bridge, lying supine with the feet on the mat and lifting the pelvis up and down from the mat, provides for movement in the spine and hips, and engages the shoulder girdle for strengthening. Patients with neck issues, certain back issues with herniated discs, osteoporosis of the spine, some types of hip replacements, and pregnancy may want to avoid this posture. In bridge, I prefer snuggling the shoulder blades closer to the spine while bending the elbows, so that the fingers point up to the sky. Then, by pressing firmly into the elbows, the scapulae and arms take most of the body weight, rather than the thoracic spine, especially when lifting the pelvis off of the floor.

Inversions in which the pelvis is higher than the head encourage the abdominal contents to shift towards the diaphragm and heart. The diaphragm then must work a bit harder during the inhalation, while the exhalation is assisted by the weight of the abdominal organs pushing towards the thoracic cavity. Normally with relaxed breathing, inhalation is active (requires work as the diaphragm contracts) while the exhalation is passive (diaphragm relaxes). Inverting the pelvis above the head, like in bridge, can strengthen the diaphragm, assuming there are no feelings of shortness of breath. Some other inversions are modified shoulder stand, standing forward folds (discussed earlier), and the more intense upward-facing wheel; each have their own unique qualities. Since this book is not intended to be a comprehensive book on asanas, the reader is encouraged to look for online images of these postures. As a caution, people who are menstruating, pregnant, have a history of retinal detachment or glaucoma, high blood pressure, heart disease, prior stroke, head or neck injury, epilepsy, or sinus issues should not perform some inversions without permission from their health care provider and close supervision.

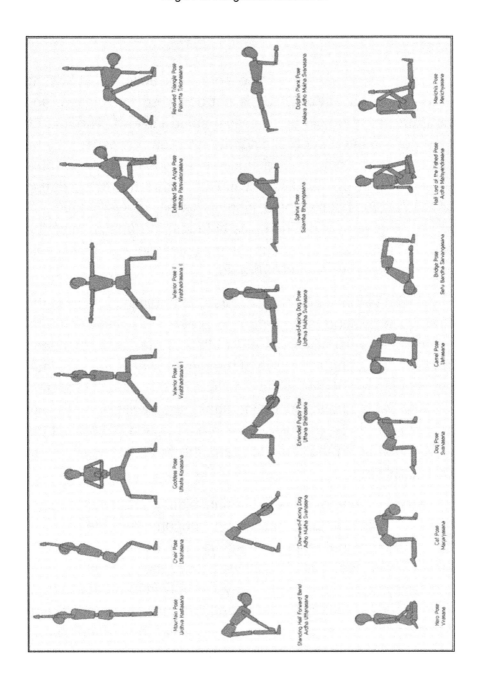

Twists

Twists are good for the spine if done correctly. Avoid twisting the lower lumbar area, which is not designed for rotation, and twist from the thoracic and cervical spine instead. The interior portion of the intervertebral disc, the nucleus pulposus, may be kept supple by twists. The nucleus pulposus is the central gelatinous part of our discs. It moves within the discs during various positions of the spine, kind of like jelly in a jelly doughnut that is being squished. The discs help support and cushion the vertebrae and prevent pressure on the spinal nerves. Twists help keep the discs mobile and hydrated.

As with virtually all yoga postures, maintaining length in the spine while twisting is important to prevent disc and vertebral compression. I usually invite elongation of the spine with each inhalation, reaching the crown of the head towards the sky, then twist with the exhalation without collapsing the spine. Untwisting a bit with each inhale, elongating again, then twisting more with each exhale can be useful to ease into a rotation. To protect the spine, avoid using the arms to crank the twist, especially in an older population.

Twists can be performed standing, sitting, side-lying, supine, or prone. Twists help compress and decompress the thoracic and intraabdominal contents, acting like a massage to the organs, intestines, the connective tissue, the lymphatics, and vascular system of the trunk. They are considered balancing to the right and left side of the body and help balance the SNS and PNS. I find it nice to do some twists both at the beginning and the end of a yoga practice. Twists connect the right and left sides of the body via the fascial connections and work synergistic groups of muscles that together produce the rotation. Pausing after releasing just one side is an enjoyable time to practice interoception, noticing the sensations arising in the body. Then progressing to doing the twist on the other side equilibrates the muscular actions and fascial connections, as well as balancing the sense of prana in the body.

Lateral Flexion of the Spine

Lateral flexion of the spine, such as crescent moon pose that involves bending to the right or left while standing, has similar benefits to twists. One side of the body is opened and stretched while the other side is compressed. The connective tissue and organs in the chest and abdomen are alternately opened or compressed. Twists provide disc and spinal movement, and the fascial connections to the extremities are lengthened. Keeping a long spine, as discussed above, applies here too.

Balancing

Balancing postures are great for the core and for building mental focus. Using the wall or a chair as a prop can be helpful in the beginning or for those with balance problems, to help gain confidence in the poses. Standing on one foot when the opportunity presents itself outside the yoga studio is a simple habit to start. Make sure you are in safe surroundings and have something to hold onto if needed. I often do this in line at the grocery store, with the cart being my handy prop. Balance is helped by picking a visual focus or "gaze" (called a *drishti*) to stare at and by exaggerating your exhale, keeping the core muscles engaged. It is the effort that counts, not the end posture. If you lose balance, just try again!

When balancing, invite attention to the quivering of core muscles and deep belly, with the intent of building their strength and stability. Embrace and encourage the effort as these muscles tend to get lazy in our chair-sitting society. Safe balance poses are a valuable tool for yoga therapists to use, especially when working with seniors. As hip fractures are a common cause of morbidity and mortality, practicing safe balancing is even more important to practice with aging to help prevent falls. Learning balances can help us practice humility, have fun, and try to release the ego.

Benefits of Asana Practice

The main way to assess if an asana is beneficial is to feel its effects, both during the posture and afterwards. Pausing for a few breaths while in a posture, and again after coming out, allows you to experience afferent sensations and builds mindfulness. Pausing is especially helpful between postures that are done on first one side and then the other. Building self-awareness physically may expand to mental and spiritual self-awareness, if given time and practice. I also encourage entering and exiting postures slowly, as the transitions are as important as the actual postures. Injuries can occur when people lose their focus on the body while moving between postures. The effects noted a day or two after a practice are also helpful in assessing what was beneficial. Yoga should be considered an exploration of yourself, including your response to the asanas.

Strengthening, stretching, and balancing are the musculoskeletal system benefits from practicing yoga. Range of motion of the joints maintains mobility needed for the activities of daily living, distributing synovial fluid (joint fluid) for healing and nourishment to the articular cartilage lining the joints. Strengthening makes you feel better and may help with daily functioning. Balancing postures promote core strength, concentration, coordination, and may help prevent falls. Besides the musculoskeletal system, yoga asanas provide respiratory, immune, cardiovascular, gastrointestinal, and psychiatric benefits, as well as others. Asanas can be considered a holistic form of exercise.

The fascia is an important integral part of the brain-body connection. Fascia, part of our connective tissue, is a three-dimensional net or web extending virtually everywhere in the body down to the cellular level. It provides structure and communication, connecting all parts of the body. Fascia is said to have six-to-ten times more sensory nerve endings than muscle. Fasciitis, or inflammation of the fascia, is known to be exquisitely painful, such as in conditions like peritonitis or necrotizing fasciitis. I believe that fascia provides pleasurable sensation too, such as the feeling after releasing a posture and the residual "ah" effect. In my mind, the fascia is like a peripheral brain, helping to explain meridians, nadis, acupuncture, and referred pain. More research is being devoted to the fascinating nature and function of fascia and connective tissue. Asanas help keep the fascia hydrated and supple.

As an aside, another interesting ongoing field of study is epigenetics, the study of how behavior can affect the expression of your genes. Epigenomes are chemical compounds that surround DNA and modify the DNA's expression or function. Epigenomes are inherited along with our DNA, but unlike DNA can be modified or changed by behavior. Epigenomes work by various mechanisms, such as adding or removing chemical groups to DNA, or wrapping DNA around proteins (known as histones). These adjustments affect the ability of proteins to "read" the gene and express it.

You may have a certain gene that programs for an effect—say, developing a certain type of cancer—but the epigenome acts like a gatekeeper to block that effect, effectively blocking the gene expression. Though your genes do not change during your lifetime, the epigenomes can be changed by behavior. If you choose healthy habits like proper diet and exercise (yoga asanas), epigenomes may keep "bad" genes, such as cancer-causing genes, turned off. Conversely, poor habits like smoking, being sedentary, and poor food choices are more likely to change the epigenome so that the "bad" gene can raise its ugly head. Epigenomes help explain how behavior directly affects health.

A small pilot study looked at 28 women reporting psychological distress and enrolled them in twice weekly yoga classes for eight weeks, then measured epigenome inflammatory markers, comparing their levels with controls.[xliii] The results did show beneficial effects on these markers in the yoga group versus the controls, though future studies are needed for verification.

In this chapter, I have shared my own tips for asanas based on my experience and training. Once again, finding a professionally trained, well-informed, empathetic teacher or yoga therapist is the best way to get started in yoga. Group classes can be beneficial with their camaraderie and the bonding experience with classmates. Most people are there with the intent and desire to improve themselves, and friendships often develop. Hopefully, the instructors also introduce some of the concepts of yoga discussed in earlier chapters, such as the yamas and niyamas, the chakras, the koshas, and pranayama.

Once comfortable with techniques and proper alignment, solo practice is wonderful too. Practicing the asanas develops muscle memory, like learning to swim or ride a bike. Eventually you may not have to think about how to do the physical postures, and your awareness is free to explore the body and breath while moving in and out of the asanas, noticing the mental, emotional, and spiritual effects of the practice. This internal awareness and exploration make yoga unique compared with most forms of exercise.

"If you go to a master to study and learn the techniques, you diligently follow all the instructions the master puts upon you. But then comes the time for using the rules in your own way and not being bound by them...You can actually forget the rules because they have been assimilated. You are an artist. Your own innocence now is of one who has become an artist, who has been, as it were, transmuted.... You can't have creativity unless you leave behind the bounded, the fixed, all the rules."

~ Joseph Campbell

Chapter Eight:
Pranayama

"Your breathing should flow gracefully, like a river, like a watersnake crossing the water, and not like a chain of rugged mountains or the gallop of a horse. To master our breath is to be in control of our bodies and minds. Each time we find ourselves dispersed and find it difficult to gain control of ourselves by different means, the method of watching the breath should always be used."

> ~ Thich Nhat Hanh (2016). "The Miracle of Mindfulness, Gift Edition" Beacon Press

Pranayama is the study and/or control of the breath. Like asanas, distinctive styles of breathing have different effects on the autonomic nervous system. When performing pranayama, you should never have a sense of air hunger or faintness. The goal is to experience the effects of the different breath techniques, not to have a breath-holding contest! Of the many different breathing techniques in yoga, some are contraindicated in certain conditions such as high blood pressure, seizures, pregnancy, glaucoma, and cardiovascular disease, as they are too activating.

The ANS, as previously mentioned, is not generally under conscious control. The ANS governs the gastrointestinal, endocrine, urinary, cardiovascular, and respiratory systems, requiring no effort by the thinking brain. While the breath is normally under control of the ANS, breathing can be controlled on a conscious level as well, making it unique among ANS functions.

When we are under stress, the SNS sends instructions to the body to breathe in specific ways. When we are crying, for example, we often exhibit a staccato type of inhalation. Chest breathing, breath holding, rapid rates, and short shallow breaths are also associated with the SNS stimulation. In chest breathing, the belly muscles are typically kept tight instead of relaxing with inhalation, and ribcage expansion alone allows for the incoming breath volume. The increased pressure from the tight belly is transmitted back up to the chest and neck, causing increased work for our diaphragm to lower with inhalation, and the use of accessory respiratory muscles like the intercostals, sternocleidomastoids, and scalenes.

Conversely, a parasympathetic "belly breath" lets the belly muscles relax and expand during inhalation along with chest expansion. This relaxation of the belly compensates for the increasing pressure of the lowered diaphragm as the lung volume expands, allowing the intra-abdominal pressure to be lower compared to when the abdominal muscles are held tight. Less work and effort are required from the diaphragm and respiratory muscles, so we feel more relaxed.[xliv] Belly breathing also provides a massaging action to the contents of the abdomen and chest, as the diaphragm is given the freedom to lower more with each inbreath, rhythmically massaging the organs. Yoga teachers use belly breathing as a foundational tool. Learning this technique can be the first step in learning to breathe in yoga.

Unless one is congested, the breath should be through the nose for warmth and humidification of the air, as well as to activate the *pingala* and *ida* nadis. Increasing the exhalation ratio compared with the inhalation favors the PNS, for example inhaling to a count of four and exhaling to a count of eight.

Another way to lengthen the exhale is to put little pauses in the exhalation, as if you were pausing while stepping down the rungs of a ladder.

Bhramari, or "bee" breath, is another calming technique that involves humming, which effectively prolongs the exhale. The sound itself is soothing, especially if a low tone like the sound of a happy bee is used. Experimenting with the position of the back of the throat and tongue makes bee breath sound like a whale song. Try it now; hum while opening and closing your jaw, keeping your lips closed, and move the root of your tongue around. The sound is intensified by plugging the ears, increasing bone conduction and vibrational sensation. This vibration may also help mobilize secretions in the sinuses and inner ears. I like to cover my eyes with cupped hands while the thumbs plug my ears. This is an example of *pratyahara*, withdrawal of the senses (visual and external sounds), which increases the internal focus on the effects of bee breath.

Alternate-nostril breath involves breathing in one nostril and switching to the other nostril at the top of each inhale, completing the breath by exhaling through the second nostril. The process is then repeated by breathing in the second nostril, then out through the first. This sequence continues for however long is desired, though there are other variations. The thumb and ring finger may be used to occlude the nostrils. The breath can be continued in a relaxed manner for as long as is comfortable. Alternate-nostril breathing can also be done as a visualization without using the fingers to plug the nostrils. This pranayama is thought to balance the PNS and SNS branches of the ANS. It also aerates the sinus areas and nasal passages, which may help during allergy seasons.

In yoga, traditionally the left nostril is cooling/soothing to breathe through, correlating with the left-sided *ida* discussed earlier in the chapter on chakras and *nadis*. Breathing through the right nostril is thought to be energizing, stimulating the right-sided *pingala*. The *ida* exits the body through the left nostril, and the *pingala* through the right. Choosing to breathe through the left nostril may be calming in nature and breathing through the right nostril may help with alertness. Our nasal passages may naturally switch dominance, with one side being more open at various times throughout the day and night. It is interesting to notice if you are feeling more relaxed when the left side is more open, versus more alert when the right nostril is.

A study on twenty-one male volunteers showed that breathing through only the right nostril increased systolic, diastolic, and mean blood pressure during a thirty-minute pranayama practice. Left nostril breathing decreased systolic and mean blood pressure, and alternate nostril breathing decreased both systolic and diastolic blood pressure.[xlv] These results correlate with the discussion on the roles of the *pingala* (activating) and *ida* (relaxing) discussed above.

Sympathetic tone, the relative amount of SNS activity, is increased by lengthening the duration of inhalation. Normally, the exhalation is longer than inhalation, so lengthening of the inbreath should be done carefully. Feeling light-headed or breathless are symptoms to avoid, and normal breathing should be resumed. Inviting the inhalation to be about the same length as the exhalation is usually enough. Noticing the effect of the practice will help you to find your beneficial duration of inbreath, so that you feel more energized but not anxious. Remember that pranayama is a practice, not a contest, and you should never feel anxious, dizzy, or short of breath.

A type of cooling breath to lower body heat is called *sitali*. The tongue is curled into a "u" shape like a straw and breathing is done with an open mouth. The air passes over the curled tongue, cooling the breath via evaporation so that cooler air enters the lungs. *Sitali* can be done on both the inhale and exhale, or the exhale can be through the nose to keep the tongue moist. The latter breath brings in the cooler outside air while getting rid of warmer air from the lungs. Either technique is good to relieve overheating, just as a dog pants through a gaping mouth when hot. However, do not pant rapidly, just breathe at a comfortable rate.

Ujjayi breath involves slightly narrowing the vocal cord opening to produce a whispering type of breath, typically done on both the inhalation and exhalation, sounding like gentle waves at a beach. The narrowing of the opening can slow the breathing rate and can provide an auditory focus for mindfulness. During an active asana class, *ujjayi* can enhance the effort of the abdominal muscles. Since the lung's air is being exhaled against the resistance of the narrowed vocal cords, the abdominal muscles tend to work harder to overcome this resistance. This engagement of the abdominal muscles provides more support to the spine and pelvis. The higher volume of air being retained in the lungs causes increased pressure in the chest, which in turn is transmitted to the abdominal cavity if the abdominal muscles are kept engaged. Thus, the spine and pelvis receive support, like putting on a girdle. The retention of air in the lungs also helps keep the airways from collapsing in conditions such as asthma and may provide for longer oxygen-carbon dioxide exchange in the lungs. *Ujjayi* breath effectively may work like pursed lip exhalation, taught by respiratory therapists for asthma and bronchial conditions to assist with keeping the airways open.

Moving in and out of yoga postures is typically coordinated with the breath in many types of yoga, such as vinyasa or ashtanga styles. Backbends and coming up from a forward fold are usually initiated while inhaling, while going into a forward fold or lateral bend are done while one is exhaling. Backbends and inhalation are both activating, while forward folds and exhalation both tend to relax the nervous system.

Emotional states are associated with various styles of breathing. For example, anxiety can stimulate the SNS, causing hyperventilation, breath holding, and shallow or variable breathing, such as when crying. Most of the pranayama described above favor the PNS and are calming in nature. Parasympathetic breath techniques have been shown to increase heart rate variability and cardiac-vagal baroreceptor tone, which are beneficial effects.[xlvi] Heart rate variability (HRV) is the difference in the time between different pairs of heart beats. Higher HRV reflects a heathier cardiovascular system and a better ability to manage physiological stress, compared to a low HRV.

Studies have shown numerous beneficial effects from relaxing styles of pranayama, such as decreased blood pressure and heart rate,[xlvii] helping depression in the elderly,[xlviii] stress reduction, and improved cognitive function.[xlix] A review of scientific evidence also shows benefits with smoking cessation, pain perception, stress and anxiety in students, pulmonary function in diseases such as asthma and TB, and reducing cancer-related symptoms.[l]

If the proper technique is chosen, pranayama is a valuable tool for union of body, mind, and spirit. Styles described above are practical, easy to learn, and readily available. One can see how these practices have great potential as part of integrative medicine. The techniques should be taught under the guidance of an experienced teacher, and some of the pranayama techniques are not appropriate for certain conditions. For example, *ujjayi* breath may be too intense for some people with some respiratory problems or may trigger mental distress in those with psychiatric issues. Two types of pranayama that are very activating, *kapalabhati* and *bhastrika*, have several contraindications and should be done with supervision, so will not be further described here.

Bandhas

The *bandhas* are muscular engagements that function as pressure gauges to control the energy of the breath and prana. Instead of the breath flowing naturally, the action of the bandhas is to block the usual direction of the flow of prana or breath and direct this energy elsewhere. Engaging *bandhas* will typically produce more energy and heat in the body as well as intensifying internal awareness. When the *bandhas* are released, energy is felt to flood more freely through the nadis that had been blocked. *Bandhas* can be used on the inhalation or exhalation, depending on the *bandha* and the goal. I recommend learning and practicing the *bandhas* under the guidance of an experienced teacher. The practice of engaging *bandhas* may have certain contraindications such as heart disease, ulcers, hernias, glaucoma, high or low blood pressure, pregnancy, menses, and recent abdominal surgery. In addition, doing this without the guidance of a good teacher may be too activating and potentially cause mental and physiological distress.

The three *bandha*s are the *mula bandha*, the *uddiyana bandha*, and the *jalandhara bandha*. *Mula bandha* is associated with the root chakra and is engaged by lifting the perineum, or pelvic floor. At first people tend to use the sphincter muscles to engage this bandha, but with practice, they learn to use the perineal body—a muscular area in front of the anus—and the pelvic floor muscles. Engaging *mula bandha* is a little like practicing Kegel exercises. This lifting of the root is believed in yoga to stop the flow of energy downward and out (*apana vayu*) and instead help it rise (*udana vayu*) through the central canal of the *sushuma*. In yogic terms, this is felt to help with the flow of prana through the chakras and *sushuma*.

Engaging this *bandha* is helpful in balance poses. One feels lighter on the feet with the upward instead of downward movement of energy. This practice also tones the pelvic floor muscles and may help with incontinence, sexual function, and excretory function. It should be noted that the pelvic floor muscles should also be allowed to relax between practicing the *bandha* and not be held in constantly. Otherwise, chronic tightness and spasms of the anatomical structures could develop, causing problems such as vaginismus (painful sex) or difficulty voiding.

Uddiyana bandha is engaged by lifting the lower abdominal muscles up and in towards the back of the heart. It is practiced at the end of an exhalation and before the inhalation. This muscular action produces a hollowing under the ribcage as energy is pulled in and up. Combining the two actions of *mula bandha* and *uddiyana bandha* engages the core muscles, including the abdominal and pelvic floor muscles, and helps maintain stability when practicing balancing postures. More internal heat and energy may be sensed rising from our root chakra area and spreading upwards. In yoga, this upward flow of prana helps cleanse the nadis, like water running through a hose helps flush out debris.

The third *bandha, jalandhara,* or "chin lock," is meant to keep the breath or prana from escaping up and out past the nose and throat, as normally happens with exhalation. *Jalandhara* is typically done after inhaling, then briefly holding the breath. The chin is tucked toward the sternal notch while drawing the chin in, and simultaneously lifting the sternum and chest up. The tongue is placed on the roof of the mouth. By pausing exhalation, upward energy, or *udana*, is effectively prevented from being transmitted out of the body. After a comfortable period of breath holding, the lock is then released with a gentle exhale. Those with high blood pressure, heart disease, and certain neck problems should avoid this *bandha. Jalandhara* is said to stimulate the thyroid and thymus area and activates the throat chakra. The muscular effect is toning of the neck flexors and stretching of the neck extensors. The practice is felt to cleanse the *nadis* in the neck region.

After mastering each bandha, all three may be combined sequentially during an exhale to produce the *maha bandha*, or the great seal. The upward energy from the *mula bandha* and *uddiyana bandha* combines with the energy from the *jalandhara* to move the energy up to the third eye and crown chakras. In Tantric yoga, the *maha bandha* is felt to awaken the kundalini, latent energy at the base of the spine, in order to rise up the *sushumna*. The benefits are said to revitalize the body, slow aging, balance the endocrine system, soothe anger, and calm the mind. This advanced practice should only be done with proper training and experience, only be held for a brief time without strain, and should be interspersed with normal periods of breathing between rounds.

Perhaps the most difficult pranayama of all to perform is simply observing the breath without letting the mind control it. As soon as the attention is turned to the breath, the mind wants to interfere with it, making the nature of the breath artificial or unnatural. This interference is normal in the beginning. With practice, this mental control is loosened, and the body can "breathe you," as it does naturally when not paying close attention to it. Watching the breath can be a form of self-study by observing the present style of breathing. Do you notice chest breathing or breath-holding because you are under stress? Can you relax into a belly breath to release this stress? When relaxed, the breath can be peaceful as a meditative focus, staying mindful of the present moment, and help release distractions or thoughts of the past and future. Combining breath awareness with observation of the heartbeat is a beautiful meditative practice of staying in the present moment.

"Being aware of your breath forces you into the present moment - the key to all inner transformation. Whenever you are conscious of the breath, you are absolutely present. You may also notice that you cannot think and be aware of your breathing. Conscious breathing stops your mind."

~ Eckhart Tolle

"I am grateful for what I am and have. My thanksgiving is perpetual. It is surprising how contented one can be with nothing definite - only a sense of existence... My breath is sweet to me..."

~ Henry David Thoreau

Chapter Nine:
Meditation

"The most common ego identifications have to do with possessions, the work you do, social status and recognition, knowledge and education, physical appearance, special abilities, relationships, person and family history, belief systems, and often nationalistic, racial, religious, and other collective identifications. None of these is you."

~ *The Power of Now: A Guide to Spiritual Enlightenment* by Eckhart Tolle, 2004

The last four steps on the eightfold path of Patanjali's *Yoga Sutras* are *pratyahara, dharana, dhyana, and samadhi*. These four steps can be conceptualized as stepping-stones along the path of meditation. *Pratyahara* is broadly defined as "withdrawal of the senses," *dharana* as "concentration," *dhyana* as "contemplation," and *samadhi* as "absorption" or "bliss." Please refer to the end of Chapter Three for further explanation of these terms. Meditation is meant to induce mental calmness, physical relaxation, help cope with illness, and improve overall health. In yoga meditation is also the path to enlightenment and *samadhi*.

Meditation typically is done in a quiet location with minimal distractions and in a comfortable body position, such as sitting, lying down, or even walking. A focus, if chosen, may be the breath, a sensation or emotion, a word or phrase, an object, or an imagery scene. Keeping an open non-judgmental attitude during the practice is important, noticing distractions and then trying to let those thoughts or sensations go without reacting to them.

Meditation may help reduce anxiety, fatigue, depression, high blood pressure, and insomnia. Studies have found it beneficial in helping symptoms of heart disease, irritable bowel and ulcerative colitis, cancer, and pain. These benefits may be gradual in onset and become more noticeable with continuation of the practice. Patients with certain psychiatric conditions rarely may find worsening of symptoms and should speak to their health care provider for referral to an experienced instructor.[li]

With many different techniques available and the constant change happening in our lives, meditation can be considered a practice that is never experienced quite the same way twice. Keeping the body absolutely still is not necessary, and some may find a moving meditation easier, especially if feeling restless. That said, stillness favors the calmness of the parasympathetic branch and can help the "mud" settle. By mud, I mean both external sensory distractions and internal mental distractions, including the ubiquitous thoughts that keep popping up and trying to take you somewhere else. My personal experience is that it takes about ten to fifteen minutes for my mud to settle.

Think of a pond with a silty bottom that is being disturbed by something, such as a dog walking through it. The silt will start floating around in the pond, making it murkier. With removal of the disturbance, in this case the movement of the dog, the mud slowly settles to the bottom, eventually leaving the water clear. So, too, can your mind become clear and undisturbed by practicing meditation and resisting distractions (represented by the dog). With practice you learn to not follow mental disturbances, but instead to let them pass, let the mud settle, and experience the clarity of a focused mind.

"Let the waters settle and you will see the moon and the stars mirrored in your own being."

~ Rumi

Meditation Techniques

Relaxing your body is a good place to start when initiating a meditation practice. If physically tense, one helpful technique is progressive muscular relaxation. This is performed by sequentially contracting and holding different muscle groups tense for several seconds, followed by releasing the muscles to a relaxed state. Another way to relax the body is to imagine breathing into various parts of your body, letting your awareness suggest warmth and heaviness while releasing tension with exhalations. The breath should be calming, such as a belly breath, as the senses are withdrawn (*pratyahara*) from your outside world. Closing the eyes, softening the gaze, or focusing on a visual object such as a candle helps prevent visual distractions.

As the body relaxes, hopefully the mind follows; relaxing the body helps the mind relax too. Meditation can be remarkably difficult, because our "monkey mind" is programmed for constant chatter. Just as your body can be twitchy, so too can your mind be restless. The mind may jump from thought to thought, like a monkey jumping from branch to branch. Training the mind to be still may be done with *dharana*, concentrating on one or two objects of choice. When you notice distractions, let them go without latching on to them or judging the fact that you had a distraction, and then refocus on your object of choice.

One lady told me she found the monkey mind metaphor, discussed in the *Upanishads*, helpful in itself as an imagery focus. She envisioned a monkey jumping from tree to tree, then imagined holding the monkey on her lap in a soothing way to calm it down. When she noticed mental distractions represented by the jumping monkey, she returned her focus to the visual image of stroking the monkey to calm herself. Another imagery technique is to think of distractions as being thought bubbles that appear in the mind, which you then choose to let dissolve or float away. Just keep redirecting your attention back to your object of focus—such as the breath, a silent repeated word, or visual image—in a non-judgmental way. Though this is a simple approach, it takes time to build up the ability to sustain attention on the object of focus. Regular practice will bear the fruit over time.

Focused-attention meditation (concentration) may be easier if two objects are picked to focus on, ideally one of them being the breath. Counting the exhalations is a straightforward way to start, so the focus is on the number of breaths as well as the feel of the breath itself. Some people prefer silently repeating a word, a phrase, or a prayer. Transcendental meditation uses this technique, repeating a mantra for 15-20 minutes twice a day. Imagery also is an option as a focus, such as imagining oneself in place or situation that is calming or healing. Other focal choices may be positive emotions such as gratitude, compassion, or loving-kindness. Visual techniques like candle gazing or focusing on a mandala (a geometric image) are also effective. The breath and heartbeat are excellent choices for me, with their ongoing rhythmic movements in my body. Nothing is more immediate and in the present moment than the breath and heartbeat.

With practice, the meditation journey may progress along the path to *dhyana*, when distractions are no longer a problem and one is more contemplative, without having to continually refocus. *Dhyana* in turn may lead to moments of becoming totally immersed or absorbed in the present meditative state, and to the trancelike state of *samadhi* as discussed in Chapter Three.

Mindfulness

Mindfulness, associated with the Buddhist tradition as a practice towards insight and enlightenment, is broadly defined as being aware of the present moment in a non-judgmental manner. Mindfulness can be a transient state of mind or be developed into a more enduring quality or trait. In the United States, Jon Kabat-Zinn, founder of Mindfulness-Based Stress Reduction, and others have advocated for mindfulness as beneficial for certain health conditions, such as chronic pain. A substantial body of evidence supports the use of mindfulness interventions in health care. Mindfulness can be described as training the attention to be in a moment-by-moment state of awareness. Practicing mindfulness in everyday life improves our ability to stay in the present moment. It also may help us to be more thoughtful in responding to life's challenges, rather than simply reacting to them. When using mindfulness as a meditation technique to gain insight into the nature of the mind, I like to use the term "open awareness."

Open awareness, also referred to as open monitoring, differs from focused attention or concentrating on an object as a meditation technique. Instead of picking something to continually refocus on, the mind is trained to remain in the present moment and observe what is happening. Sensations and thoughts are noticed then released. This can be difficult to do, as instead of releasing the thought, we are usually drawn into some storyline of a thought pattern. That thought pattern can lead into the script of a personal mini-series, in which we are usually the star. These mental scripts tend to ruminate on the past or fret about the future. Daydreams are splendid examples of this. We may even be unaware we are daydreaming until we "come to" and bring the attention back to the present moment.

Open awareness can be an informative form of self-study. Noticing getting caught up in a daydream or mind chatter is the first goal. Without judgment, see where those thoughts started to lead you, and then let go with compassion. Soon something else will try to capture the attention, and you repeat the process. What you learn about your topics and patterns of thinking can be enlightening. You can learn to recognize ruminations as they are happening and release negative *samskaras*, habitual patterns of thought. Thoughts and attention can then be redirected to the here and now.

Imagine that you are in a busy train station, sitting on a bench and noticing people. The people represent different thoughts, and the trains they are boarding represent different trains of thought. If you get on a train with someone, you become part of the thought train. The goal is to not do this, but instead to stay on the bench as the observer. Notice the thought (person), then let it go, and come back to the present moment—you on a bench noticing. Avoid letting the monkey mind draw you away from the now. Life is really a series of moments, and we should not waste our precious moments by continually fretting about the future or ruminating on the past. Instead, let us practice living in the now.

Eventually, thoughts are recognized as transient mental events. Thoughts are impermanent, changing quicker than the aging body. Practicing open awareness may be done as a meditation practice while being in stillness. Mindfulness may also be practiced with any activity, such as walking, doing housework, or having conversations. Eventually, mindfulness may be incorporated as a permeating habitual trait.

In my own personal meditation practice, I often start with the focused concentration technique, using the breath and the heartbeat to focus on. Then as I become more relaxed and in the present, I switch to open awareness. If I feel myself getting too distracted, unable to turn away from thought trains, then I switch back to the breath and heartbeat focus. I can choose to go back and forth between those two techniques depending on what kind of a day I am having in my meditation practice. It is wonderful that no two meditation practices are ever the same. The only thing constant in life is change and meditation practice reflects that.

"I am not my thoughts, emotions, sense perceptions, and experiences. I am not the content of my life. I am Life. I am the space in which all things happen. I am consciousness. I am the Now. I Am."
~ Eckhart Tolle

Studies Involving Meditation

Numerous studies have shown the benefits of yoga and meditation, some of which were discussed in Chapter Six, and I would like to mention a few others. As a reminder, there are certain contraindications or cautions for meditation with some psychiatric disorders, and a trained professional should be consulted, especially for those with a history of physical, emotional, or mental trauma.

Dr. John Denninger is the director of research at the Benson-Henry Institute for Mind Body Medicine at Massachusetts General Hospital. He and his coworkers study mind-body techniques, and a 2013 study showed that the relaxation response may switch on genes that beneficially mediate telomere maintenance, mitochondrial function, insulin secretion, and energy metabolism. At the same time, genes are switched off that are linked to the inflammatory response and stress reaction. By inducing calmness, meditation is not just affecting the mental state but also affecting the physiology of the whole body.[lii]

Recent studies on telomeres are also fascinating. Elizabeth Blackburn won the 2009 Nobel Prize in Physiology or Medicine for her work on telomere biology. Telomeres are sections at the ends of the DNA chromosomes that help keep the DNA from unraveling. Each time a cell divides, the telomeres lose a bit of length. As the telomeres get shorter, the lifespan of the cell is also shortened, translating to aging and the eventual death of the cell.[liii] Shorter telomeres are associated with decreased immune function, cardiovascular disease, Alzheimer's disease, and osteoporosis.

An enzyme called telomerase helps prevent shortening of the telomere and lengthens the life span of the cell by keeping the DNA from unraveling. In one study, women with high perceived stress levels had the equivalent of ten years of shortening of their telomeres, compared with women with low stress levels.[liv] Mindfulness and meditation, in this case used to help stress levels, were associated with increased telomerase enzyme activity, indicating longer cell life. Other studies footnoted have shown the benefits of meditation being associated with longer telomeres.[lv] [lvi] [lvii] The findings in these early studies suggest the need for further research on mind-body medicine. Meditation may eventually be considered a fountain of youth!

Encouraging appropriate patients to incorporate mind-body relaxation into their daily life could significantly decrease individual and national healthcare costs. "Relaxation Response and Resiliency Training and Its Effects on Healthcare Resources" is a retrospective, controlled observational study that looked at 4,452 patients referred to the Benson-Henry Institute for Mind Body Medicine at Massachusetts General Hospital. This intervention group underwent resiliency training in the relaxation response to decrease sympathetic tone. After training, these patients were compared to 13,149 controls by measuring billable encounters for healthcare, such as doctor appointments.

After the relaxation training intervention, the results showed a decrease in total utilization of healthcare by 43% in the trained group compared to controls during the following year.[lviii] Fewer visits to the doctor for illness and chronic medical problems reflect lower healthcare costs, and perhaps fewer prescriptions, better work productivity, and better overall health of the patients. Learning to practice relaxation, which can be done by virtually anyone, anywhere, anytime with little initial cost for training, could powerfully affect the nation's overall state of health and healthcare costs.

A study by Holzel et al (2011) was appropriately titled "Mindfulness practice leads to increases in regional brain gray matter density." MRIs were performed before and after eight weeks of training in body scanning, mindful yoga practice, and sitting meditation. The results of the MRIs showed increases in gray matter (brain cells and surrounding structures that process information) in the hippocampus, posterior cingulate, cortex, temporal-parietal, and cerebellum after mindfulness-based stress reduction practice. These areas of the brain involve emotional regulation, learning, memory, self-referencing, and perspective taking.[lix] To me, that translates to less anger and anxiety, better recall, retention of new information, and putting life's problems in perspective.

Another interesting study examined the techniques of focused attention and open monitoring, which I call open awareness.[lx] MRIs were done on both novice meditators with ten days of meditation training and experienced Buddhist monks. Executive brain function helps you reason, plan, and respond in appropriate ways to problem solving and stressors. These MRIs demonstrated activation of the executive brain function areas during meditation, a representation of self-regulation. This study also showed a beneficial functional reorganization of brain activity patterns in the practiced Buddhist mediators, occurring in the prefrontal and insular areas of the brains. Both focused attention and open-monitoring style meditation developed these parts of the brain. This activation and reorganization representing neuroplasticity may allow the higher centers of the brain to choose wisely, rather than reacting impulsively to life stressors.

As mentioned before, neuroplasticity is the brain's ability to remodel itself by creating new pathways and even new brain cells. New brain cells have been shown to grow in the hippocampus, which is active in learning and memory. Scientists used to think that the brain could not grow new cells; once brain cells were lost, they were lost for good. Researchers now know this old assumption is not true. Stroke patients who benefit from rehab are a good example of neuroplasticity.

What you do, and how you think, affects not just your thoughts but the actual anatomy and functioning of your brain. Wise choices in life can change your brain, creating new connections to reprogram yourself in a beneficial way. Just as exercise can reshape the physical body, practicing mindfulness and meditation may reshape your brain. What you practice becomes stronger with repetition.

Neuroplasticity correlates with the yoga concept of releasing *samskaras*, negative patterns of thought that do not benefit you. Doing this requires self-study (*svadhyaya*) and practice. The more you practice negativity, the more negative you become, which can spread to those around you. If instead you practice positivity in your own head and with your actions, you will become a more positive being. Not only do you benefit, but so does society around you, in effect working like a beneficial contagious virus.

"The way to overcome negative thoughts and destructive emotions is to develop opposing, positive emotions that are stronger and more powerful."

~ The Dalai Lama

Loving-Kindness

As a final note, I want to discuss loving-kindness as a meditation technique. This practice usually starts by sending loving-kindness to yourself, then to your loved ones and close friends. Next this feeling and intention is extended to casual acquaintances, and then to strangers. More difficult, you start to envision sending loving-kindness to those whom you dislike or harbor ill feelings towards. Finally, loving-kindness is extended out to all beings. I like to end with circling back to myself as both the giver and receiver.

After practicing loving-kindness meditation for some time, it is interesting to notice how interactions change with people, especially those who were in the category of being disliked. Recalling the practice causes the intention of kindness to enter your mind, which may be reflected in your body language in subtle ways, as well as in your conversations. Mirroring is the subconscious mimicking of another person's gestures, attitudes, and body language. The person with whom you had a grudge picks up on your kinder body language and starts to mirror you. There appears to be a mutual "melting" of aggression and ill-feelings. Instead, that person starts being kinder too. The positivity of loving-kindness is truly contagious.

Loving-kindness is a type of Buddhist meditation called metta. "Metta" means positive energy and kindness. Your heart feels more open to positive emotions, compassion, and kindness, increasing empathy towards all others and towards yourself. Interestingly, metta is the meditation technique most likely to evolve into a character trait in a relatively brief period of time. This was discussed in Chapter Six under the section "EEGs, State of Consciousness, and Meditation" in the study involving long-term Buddhist meditators. As mentioned, a character trait is a lasting habitual way of acting or thinking, in contrast to just a temporary state of mind. Humans are social creatures, and it seems we are wired or programmed for loving-kindness to be the most accessible meditative technique that promotes true changes in behavior.[lxi] Practicing loving-kindness not only improves you as a person but benefits society. Just think what a better world it might be if everybody practiced this meditation.

"Anger is an acid that can do more harm to the vessel in which it is stored than to anything on which it is poured."

~ Mark Twain

"As a single footstep will not make a path on the earth, so a single thought will not make a pathway in the mind. To make a deep physical path, we walk again and again. To make a deep mental path, we must think over and over the kind of thoughts we wish to dominate our lives."

~ Henry David Thoreau

"If you don't love yourself, you cannot love others. You will not be able to love others. If you have no compassion for yourself then you are not able of developing compassion for others."

~ The Dalai Lama

Chapter Ten:
Integrating Yoga with Western Medicine

The testimonial below is from a lovely woman, Marilyn McSpadden, who has practiced yoga for many years. I have had the pleasure of leading a community yoga group that she and her husband attend for over ten years. Friendships and camaraderie often develop when people practice yoga together, as has happened within this group.

"I have been practicing yoga for almost 14 years now. Although the beauty of yoga poses always were appealing to me, my motivation for getting started was to counteract the sore and stiff muscles I was starting to experience at age 50...Ironically, the first yoga I experienced is what I would call "gym yoga." Our teacher was very young, and we did the same "yoga routine" every class. But even with a lack of teaching expertise, something profound started happening, I felt more in touch and aware of my body than I ever had in my life. I left every class with a sense of physical well-being and calm. I had always carried a lot of tension in my shoulders and neck, and this almost entirely disappeared, along with periodic tension headaches. My arms and shoulders became toned without resorting to lifting weights, and the muscle stiffness I was starting to experience in mid-life was lessening. I was on my way to a permanent practice.

"By focusing on my breath and releasing any thoughts during my practice, I have gained more awareness of and control over my thinking. This has been revolutionary for me, helping me do such disparate things as to sleep better, stop multi-tasking, put down electronics, focus on the person in front of me, pray, and just be more aware of negative thought patterns as I seek to replace them with acceptance and grace towards others and myself.

"Yoga has also helped me address something I have always struggled with—achieving a balance between all the many and often competing demands of life: work, home, health, relationships, hobbies, and service. I have to say a healthy balance is always a work in progress, but yoga has helped me clarify my values and make choices to live more in tune with them."

Reproduced with the kind permission of Marilyn McSpadden

The above beautifully written testimonial reflects what I often hear from people who have chosen to embrace and practice yoga. I am amazed at how quickly new students start to notice the difference in how they feel when attending group classes routinely. I find these beneficial effects to be almost universally true.

However, some people need more individualized attention because of ongoing issues or medical conditions. A yoga therapist can prove particularly helpful for these people. Yoga therapists collaborate with a client on an individual basis or work with groups of people who have similar issues. The profession of yoga therapy is relatively new in the West but is being embraced as a holistic supplement to Western medical care and can be a valuable addition to integrative health.

One of the goals of this book is to help health professionals and clients (patients) understand what yoga is and how it works. I wanted to describe the concepts, tools, and techniques a yoga therapist uses, as for example in the chapter on the doshas. I believe a yoga therapist can augment the skill sets of physical therapy, occupational therapy, respiratory therapy, and spiritual counselors to promote holistic integrated care. Back in my life as a physician, I would have loved to have access to consultation with a yoga therapist to promote wellness and bring comfort to my patients, especially those in a hospital setting or for end-of-life issues.

If you have ever been in the hospital, you know hospitalization tends to not be very conducive for rest and recuperation. Someone is always coming to draw blood or to poke, prod, ask questions, or take you somewhere for a test. You may have an IV or other tubes with flashing lights and alarms going off, not to mention sleeping in a strange place, perhaps with a roommate, instead of home in your own bed. Your loved ones may not be present. Add to this the stress of being sick, not feeling well, or having frightening tests done, and you can see how a hospital setting may challenge the ability to rest and heal.

Now imagine if a yoga therapist came into the hospital room with the intent of helping you feel better and give you a "time-out" from stressors. Having assessed your history from medical records, techniques would be offered that are appropriate for your needs. Considerations by the yoga therapist may also include assessing your dosha type (Chapter Four), the energy level of the *koshas* (Chapter Five), and which areas of the body relating to chakras (Chapter Six) may need attention. Tools offered from asana, pranayama, meditation, and spiritual practices would be guided by the therapist's assessment, using techniques to decrease stress level and aid the healing process.

Recall the visual image from Chapter Six of the two snakes and the staff in the caduceus symbol used by medical associations. To me, the caduceus image can also be used to represent yoga therapy as part of integrative medicine. The two intertwining snakes can be equated with Western medicine and yoga therapy, with the staff being the individual or patient. I like to think of the Western medical system as being more aligned with the *pingala nadi:* SNS-activating, heating, action-oriented, detailed thinking, left-brain function; whereas yoga and ayurvedic medicine represent the *ida nadi:* PNS-activating, cooling, restful, holistic, right-brain function. In allegorical yogic terms, the *pingala* (Western) and *ida* (yoga therapy) communicate and merge in the intelligent perception of the third-eye chakra (wise therapeutic choices) to keep the energy of the *sushumna* open, representing optimal health of the patient.

The following is a case study written by my daughter, Kelsey Kraemer, which demonstrates the cooperation of these two systems in a hospital setting. Kelsey is a certified yoga therapist and has experience helping hospitalized patients who have complex medical issues. The medical terminology may be a bit technical for some, but I think all readers can appreciate this case study as an example of the benefits of holistic care. I envision yoga therapy becoming a profession commonly found in hospital settings, incorporating stress reduction and coping techniques to promote healing and recuperation.

Yoga Therapy as Part of Integrative Care for Complex Patient

Kelsey Kraemer, MS, C-IAYT, E-RYT500

This case study is of a patient who is a 47-year-old female on inpatient service presenting with Crohn's disease and enterocutaneous fistulas. Previous medical history includes malignant neoplasm of the bladder. Patient presents with significant anterior and posterior open trunk wounds. Patient's physical therapy goals include increased length of time tolerating the cardiac chair in physical therapy treatment, with the goal of her standing and eventually walking. Patient was referred to yoga therapy concurrent with physical therapy to help manage the patient's anxiety during physical therapy treatment. Patient is limited during physical therapy [PT] and yoga therapy by obesity, pain, and anxiety. She experiences high levels of anxiety prior to PT treatments, reporting she is afraid of feeling pain and of the chance of falling. The yoga therapy protocol for this patient was developed to activate the parasympathetic nervous system, decrease the patient's pain intensity, and alleviate symptoms of anxiety that occur surrounding her physical therapy appointments. The interventions used cultivated interoception and integrated spiritual practices to bring about eudaimonia. Interventions included breath awareness, guided visualization, and mantra.

Throughout four weeks of treatment, the patient was administered two weekly surveys, the University of Washington Resilience Scale and a four question survey created by the yoga therapist. Patient reports experiencing increased resilience, decreased anxiety, and decreased perceived pain when she received yoga therapy with physical therapy as opposed to physical therapy alone.

Yoga Therapy was effective for increasing resilience, decreasing anxiety and pain level during physical therapy treatment. Yoga therapy may be a beneficial complementary practice for complex conditions and as part of intensive hospital integrative care. Yoga may be an essential part of integrative care to decrease anxiety and pain as part of other medical care.

Thanks to Kelsey Kraemer for sharing this case study and her contributions to the development of the profession of yoga therapy.

In addition to individual sessions, clients or patients may benefit from group classes that are composed of individuals with similar issues. Incorporating a shared socialization time before or after a group class allows therapeutic bonding among people experiencing similar stressors. Examples include cancer,

Parkinson's disease, PTSD, fibromyalgia, prenatal and postnatal yoga, heart disease, low-back problems, and chronic pain. The yoga teacher or yoga therapist should be well versed in which tools and modifications are appropriate for each group. Modifications should be offered for different capabilities, and clients should be encouraged to "opt out" if something does not feel right for them.

It is helpful for the yoga therapist to explain how to determine if something may not be appropriate for an individual. People new to yoga practices may have difficulty paying close enough attention to bodily sensations, and may not know when to back off or opt out of a pose. Pain, numbness, tingling, shortness of breath, or any physical or emotional distress are signs to stop or modify the practice. Close monitoring by the yoga therapist is essential, who can observe for signs of discomfort such as grimacing, strained facial expressions, breath holding, or misalignment.

Clients may also be referred to yoga therapists for outpatient individual sessions. A referral from a health professional ideally includes the applicable diagnoses, goals, and any restrictions or contraindications. A full intake evaluation by the yoga therapist includes chief complaints, diagnoses, goals, medications, past medical history, lifestyle habits, and social support system. Assessment of the posture, gait, movement, and breathing patterns is typically done. The doshas and koshas may be evaluated to help guide the choices of yogic tools. The goal is to address the client's physical, mental, emotional, and spiritual needs.

The client typically is given a program to practice at home in addition to the sessions with the therapist. Usually, several sessions are needed with the clients to incorporate proper breath work, teach alignment in physical postures, get feedback, and introduce other teachings of yoga, including meditation techniques when appropriate.

When I see clients for a yoga therapy session, I try to consider both their goals and their attitude towards yoga. Some people may want asana practices and some breath work, but nothing "woo-woo." Others may be open to the idea of meditation, energy centers, and other yogic concepts. Practices are incorporated gradually, building onto prior sessions while trying to meet the client's wants and needs. I like to recommend supplemental reading material to those who are interested in learning more about the teachings of yoga, helping to enrich subsequent sessions for the informed client. This also allows the clients to help choose concepts and techniques that are beneficial for self-care as part of an ongoing individual yoga practice when sessions have ended.

Teaching a client how to pay attention to physical sensations and mental responses is an important first step to guide the therapeutic process. The yoga therapist encourages interoception (awareness of sensations arising within the body) and introspection while clients are trying a posture, breath, or meditative technique by asking the client to tune in to how they feel, both during and after the technique. If a pleasant glow is experienced, then things are on the right track. The following are some guidelines yoga therapists use to achieve various effects and to help guide therapeutic choices.

Asanas/Postures (Chapter Seven)

Relaxing Asanas: forward folds, restorative and yin-style yoga using props, slow-paced, any comfortable lying position

Invigorating Asanas: backbends, balance postures, holding isometric postures, faster-paced flow, standing

Asanas Balancing to Autonomic Nervous System: Mixture of backbends with forward folds, twists both directions, medium paced

Pranayama/Breath techniques (Chapter Eight)

Relaxing Pranayama: Exhalation longer than inhalation, left-nostril breathing, bee breath, belly (diaphragmatic) breath, slower rate

Invigorating Pranayama: Exhalation equal to inhalation, right-nostril breath, *bhastrika* and *kapalabhati* breath (some contraindications), chest breathing (especially with tight abdominal muscles or *uddiyana bandha*), faster rate

Cooling Pranayama: Sitali (breathing through curled tongue with mouth open)

Variable effect: Ujjayi Pranayama - gently narrowing the glottis to produce audible breath sounding like gentle waves; can be used during vigorous practice or as a meditative aide

Introducing Meditation Techniques

As previously discussed in the last chapter, meditation sessions may start with relaxing the physical body first by assuming a comfortable body position and using techniques such as progressive relaxation and a relaxing pranayama.

Concentrating on an object, the focused-type meditation, such as breath awareness, imagery, gratitude, mantra, or loving-kindness, may then be used to promote emotional and mental relaxation. Which focus to choose depends on the client goals and what appeals to the client. The therapist's assessment of the client's needs, including the energetic assessment (koshas) and dosha type, may also help guide the choice of meditation technique. Being verbally led by the therapist during meditation permits the client to learn techniques and then practice at home, using audio files or apps if needed. Introducing mindfulness as a meditation technique, by guiding awareness through the present sensations, may encourage the individual to practice mindfulness during daily activities as well.

The client should feel safe and be given permission to exit meditation if the session starts to become overwhelming in any way. Care should be taken to not introduce too much, too quickly in the first few sessions. Sometimes turning the awareness inward may dredge up traumatic memories and cause distress or panic. Turning the awareness to another focus which invites feelings of safety and calm can be used to counteract this. Examples are returning to the focus of a calming style of breath, imagining a nurturing safe place, or listening to a pleasant sound. Therapists specially trained in trauma counseling are recommended for those with moderate or severe mental health issues such as PTSD. Yoga therapists working with these groups should work in conjunction with a mental health professional.

Sequencing Components of Sessions

Sequencing in a typical group yoga class is comprised of centering (such as bringing the awareness to the breath or the present moment), intention setting, warmups, progressing to the more physically active part of class (perhaps with a peak pose), cool down, stretches, and a final relaxation or meditation time. Offering modifications of postures to accommodate each individual's strength, flexibility, and balance is important. Progression in a safe, mindful manner to more demanding variations happens over time with practice.

However, individual sessions may not include all the above components. Time may not allow for all the typical class components. The client may only need breath work, or meditation, or they may not be physically able to do asanas. Perhaps a client only wants the physical practice, though proper warm up and cool down should be done if more vigorous asanas are taught. Session components are determined by the individual's goals, ability, time, and needs.

I will now present some scenarios on how individual yoga sessions may be devised for individuals with specific medical complaints. These case studies are fictional but based on my real life experiences and are meant to highlight and demonstrate some of the topics which have been covered. The presentations are not meant to be comprehensive or detailed and are not intended to be followed as yoga therapy prescriptions. These examples represent my approach to the scenarios, which may differ from other yoga therapists' choices.

Case Study #1

A 48-year-old divorced female in good general health wants to try yoga. Her key issues are intermittent low-back pain, stress, and a 40-pound weight gain in the last five years. Her appetite is hard to control, and diet includes fast foods and too many carbohydrates. She reports no stomach or bowel complaints. She has a sedentary lifestyle except for walking two miles three times a week. Social stressors include two teenage children at home and caring for her elderly parents. Sleep is sound, though she finds it hard to get out of bed in the morning. She works part time as a receptionist where she sits most of the day. Her health history lists no other medical issues, and she is not on any medications. She describes her energy level as low and believes she may be mildly depressed. She has discussed all of the above with her doctor during a recent checkup, and they agreed yoga may be helpful. She read that yoga is good for stress and back pain, and she wants to lose weight.

This client presents with typical *kapha* dosha issues with her weight gain, overeating, tendency to be sedentary, sluggish feeling in the morning, and mild depression. Her stress, lack of exercise, and weight gain may all be contributing to her back pain. The yoga therapy exam shows low energy levels, especially in her physical body, with a slumped posture and a forward head position. Her flexibility is limited in her back and hamstrings, and she is slow getting up and down from a chair.

Mindfulness could be introduced to the client as a practice to bring awareness to her eating habits. Setting the intention to eat slowly and savor the flavor and texture of food, while honoring feelings of satiety, is a mindfulness practice. She may begin to notice if she is eating to avoid her emotions, such as feeling depressed. Eventually she may learn to recognize the mental triggers, or samskaras, that prompt her to choose "comforting" foods such as junk food and carbohydrates. She may then be able to pause and choose foods that are more suitable for her dosha type, helping to normalize her weight, and calming inflammation in the body. Using a pranayama technique to help calm the mind and body may help her to avoid binging and reduce her perceived level of stress. Examples are alternate-nostril breath, belly breath, or bee breath.

Asana practice should include some energizing backbends, incorporating proper alignment and safety cues for the spine, and in the beginning using props for easier access. Appropriate core work to help protect and strengthen the low back is important. Range of motion of the spine, pelvis, and hips would help increase mobility, ease stiffness, and promote healthy discs. With time and commitment, postures may be adjusted to be more challenging.

Stretches to help the low back include lying supine while bringing knees to chest, some gentle spinal twists, and supine hamstring stretches. A gentle supported backbend in the supine position, such as lying back over a bolster, would be good for opening the chest and increasing energy in the physical, mental, and emotional layers of the koshas. A choice for ending the physical work may be a relaxing restorative asana for the back, such as legs-up-the-wall pose, accompanied by progressive relaxation cued by the yoga therapist. A loving-kindness meditation for self-care would be nice for her, or a guided imagery to include a warm dry desert sky, in order to sooth her *kapha* dosha qualities of water and cool earth.

The advantage of an individual session is that it can be tailored to the client's needs. Issues can be identified and addressed in a way that a group class does not. The close attention of a one-on-one relationship allows for a more intimate practice and feedback adjustment. Eventually, joining a gentle or basics yoga class would be beneficial for this client and provide some needed socialization. Learning postures with proper alignment, pranayama, and mindfulness will build her confidence, strength, and flexibility along with improving the body-mind connection.

Case Study #2

A 35-year-old male runner wants to improve his flexibility with yoga, especially in his low back and hamstrings. He runs about five miles every day and rides his bike about 30 miles on weekends. His job, mainly computer work, consists of a 60-hour work week from both the home and office, and is described as stressful. Medical history is significant for high blood pressure, currently controlled by medications. He is married with two young children and his wife also works outside the home. They share household duties and child rearing. He has trouble falling asleep, sleeps about five hours a night, and states he finds it difficult to relax. He eats five to six times a day, makes healthy food choices, and has no weight issues. Alcoholic consumption is about twelve beers per week; he denies smoking or other drug use. He reports occasional heartburn, being prone to anger if something triggers him, and often feels restless or overheated. His exam shows a ruddy complexion, an intense gaze and affect, good posture and muscle tone, and some tightness in the hamstrings and low back.

This client represents a classic *pitta* dosha type with high blood pressure, anger issues, heartburn, competitive lifestyle, and difficulty falling asleep. He needs some stress reduction and a style of yoga that will allow him to unwind. Introducing centering by teaching diaphragmatic belly breathing would be a lovely place to start. Then, after warmups and a brief active practice to burn off energy and restlessness, a slower-paced asana practice may help sooth his fiery *pitta* nature. A restorative or yin yoga style would help sooth his overwrought sympathetic nervous system and provide longer stretching. Holding hamstring and back stretches for a few minutes would help increase his flexibility. Supported postures such as legs up the wall, or seated forward fold over a bolster, would provide length to the muscles and fascia of his back body and give him some time out to chill from his busy life. Final relaxation may be initiated with progressive relaxation cues for muscle groups. Cueing his awareness to the different *kosha* layers would build a deeper relaxation and mind-body connection.

A home practice of stretches after his runs may be useful as quality family time by including his children, modelling healthy behavior for them. The client may eventually enjoy a slow-paced flow or restorative group yoga class to supplement his fitness program and help with stress reduction. Meditation should be a component of his yoga practice, including self-study and practicing mindfulness of the present moment to help control anger. Imagery of being alone on a cool, quiet mountaintop would soothe his *pitta* dosha. Suggesting lifestyle changes such as hourly physical breaks from his workstation while doing some brief asana poses or using a meditation app may be helpful. Proper body and computer positioning should be discussed. As his stress level decreases, perhaps his alcohol consumption would too, helping his heartburn, lowering the blood pressure, and soothing his anger issues.

Case Study #3

A 53-year-old female diagnosed with breast cancer six months ago, treated with surgery and radiation, is referred by her family physician. She had reconstructive surgery for her mastectomy and has received her surgeon's permission to do yoga. She reports feeling tightness from scar tissue and feels "out of balance" in her chest area. The breast implant still feels "foreign" to her. She is getting physical therapy for the restricted range of motion of her shoulder. Other medical history is unremarkable, and she has a good support system, including an understanding spouse. Lifestyle includes regular exercise, eight hours of sleep per night, healthy eating habits, and rare alcohol use. She wants to take individual yoga sessions for her shoulder and to explore meditation and spirituality.

Since this client requests learning about spirituality and meditation, it would be especially appropriate to introduce some of the teachings of yoga as part of her sessions, such as the *kleshas*, the eightfold path, and the *koshas*. By recommending some suggestions for reading, she can expand her knowledge and educate herself in her own time as well. She may want to keep a journal of how yoga teachings may be applicable in her life.

The *koshas* as a teaching focus would address the various aspects of self, including the innermost core of spirituality. I usually ask clients, "How do you feel physically, energetically, mentally, emotionally, spiritually?" I allow for pauses between each layer of the *koshas* to give the client time for reflection. This form of self-study, or *svadyaya,* is intended to promote the client's self-awareness. Scanning the *kosha* layers at both the beginning and again at the end of a session demonstrates the effect of the yoga practice. Hopefully, the layers feel what I refer to as an "energized calmness" after a helpful yoga session.

Having faced a cancer diagnosis, the client expressed a desire to explore her own spirituality. An exploration of the concepts in the *kleshas,* discussed in Chapter Five, regarding ignorance of true self and embracing her spiritual core as permanent, may be of interest to her. Of course, all clients are free to choose their own belief systems, and yogic teachings should not be forced on anyone or considered a dogmatic part of yoga. The goal is to learn concepts that may bring comfort, not to impose a way of thinking that may be unhelpful or counter to a client's beliefs.

Physically, particular care should be taken with the client's shoulder and chest, keeping in mind any restrictions by the doctor. Awareness of her body sensations would be important for safety and to enhance the body-mind connection. Asanas concentrating on alignment with the liberal use of props could help rebalance her physical body after her recent cancer treatment. Shoulder work should be gentle and gradual, incorporating some restorative supported supine twists for stretching. Mindfulness enhances the physical treatment. The yoga therapist might bring the client's awareness to the movement of the breath in her surgical area and introduce the practice of self-kindness and compassion for the ongoing healing process. Incorporating meditation techniques at home, such as mindful walking in nature and practicing gratitude for the gift of the present moments may also contribute to her well-being.

Case Study #4

An 82-year-old man is recuperating from a mild stroke that occurred two months ago; his doctor has referred him for yoga therapy to help with strengthening and balance. The stroke has left the client with mild weakness of one hand and unsteadiness on his feet. He has used a walker and is progressing to a cane since his stroke, while still receiving outpatient physical therapy. He takes medications for blood pressure, cholesterol, and blood thinners. His wife is his primary caregiver and is also interested in yoga. Prior to his stroke, he walked two miles a day. He often awakens in the middle of the night and has difficulty going back to sleep. He is retired, no longer drives since his stroke, and quit smoking in his fifties. His appetite has diminished over the last few months, and he is concerned that he is losing weight, which he has discussed with his doctor. Activities he enjoys include reading, watching TV, and short walks with his walker or cane. His main concerns are the weak hand and unsteady balance. He also reports feeling anxious and worried about his health and mortality since his stroke. The yoga therapist's exam finds an anxious, thin, elderly male with poor balance, generalized weakness, and weak hand grip.

This man represents a *vata* dosha with his weight loss, sleep disturbance, anxiety, and advancing age. Initially, individual sessions are best for this client as he is at risk for fall and injury, and he has some loss of muscular control and proprioception because of his stroke. Chair yoga is fine, but he also needs to work on his balance. Blood thinners make falls more dangerous, as bleeding from injuries may be more prolonged and profuse. Standing postures should be done under close supervision to prevent falls, using props such as a chair, a wall, a corner of the room where the walls converge, or a walker. Hip fractures are a major cause of morbidity and mortality in the elderly. Improving his balance may help to reduce the likelihood of future falls and potential fractures. Asanas should also incorporate core work and range of motion of the joints. Strengthening and stretching of his weak hand and arm should be given special attention. As always, introducing various yoga breath styles such as belly breath and *ujjayi* might help increase his energy levels and respiratory function. The yoga therapist can cue him to move slowly, using pauses between position changes or before initiating ambulation, to build mindfulness. Developing a habit of taking four or five belly breaths after transitioning from supine to sitting, and again from sitting to standing, and before walking on may help him be less prone to falls.

A mental grounding practice, for example imagining heavy sand like in an hourglass pouring into his legs, may appeal when standing and working on his balance. During the end of sessions, lying down while tucked in with blankets or light sandbags may help him relax and counteract the *vata* tendencies of coolness, movement, and space. Imagining warmth, safety, and stillness, such basking on a warm sandy beach, might help to counteract the anxious restlessness of *vata*. If approved by his doctor, warm nourishing foods like stews and carbohydrates may help stimulate his appetite and prevent weight loss.

If his wife is able and willing, the yoga therapist might invite her to assist her husband with his daily yoga homework, and they could even practice together as a couple if desired. His lifestyle has undergone a dramatic change, with significant loss of autonomy and control, including not being able to drive anymore. Encouraging him to talk about his experience and journal about how the stroke has affected him may give him some insight and purpose. Noticing how the practice of yoga changes his internal dialog and recognizing negative *samskaras* may help him to focus on a more positive outlook. Encouraging him to explore his spiritual center, perhaps discussing the *kleshas*, may help decrease his fear of death. He should be advised to continue regular checkups with his physician to monitor his progress, medications, and blood pressure. After the client's practice is deemed safe, group yoga classes available for stroke survivors may be therapeutic for him and provide socialization.

"When you go through life ... it all seems accidental at the time it is happening. Then when you get on in your 60s or 70s and look back, your life looks like a well-planned novel with a coherent theme... Incidents that seemed accidental, pure chance, turn out to be major elements in the structuring of this novel. Schopenhauer says, 'Who wrote this novel? You did.'"

~ Joseph Campbell

A Personal Anecdote

I would like to share a personal powerful experience I had that shows how effective yoga therapy can be in the hospital setting. In early 2020, right before the COVID epidemic, I had the honor of substituting for my daughter Kelsey Kraemer at Simon Cancer Center's CompleteLife Program during her parental leave. I was excited to have this chance to practice my skills as a yoga therapist in an inpatient setting. Many of the patients were receiving cancer treatment or organ transplants, or they were having relapses or complications requiring hospitalization.

It was lovely to provide some moments of physical and mental relaxation to these patients. I would often help them with guided imagery and breath work, and I could see their faces and shoulders visibly relax and their heart and breath rates go down. A common technique I used was to ask them to think of a favorite place, imagine they were there, and guide them to silently visualize what they saw, heard, felt, smelled, and tasted in this place. Then they were invited to imagine holding and also being held by someone or something special, feeling the exchange of love and compassion in their heart center.

One day I was asked to see someone who required surgery for a lung problem. When I walked into the room, I realized the patient had just returned from surgery, with his nurse busy at his bedside. He was having acute surgical rib cage pain and had a chest tube in place. He was also on a ventilator, which controls the rate of breathing. The breathing tube from a ventilator is uncomfortable and feels unnatural, and a common response is for patients to try and pull it out. Though this person was medicated, he was still agitated and in pain, and was fighting the breathing tube as well as trying to pull at his chest tube. Because he was intubated, he was unable to speak but was alert enough to communicate by gesturing. After asking permission and if he wanted to see me, both the patient and his nurse waved me in.

I usually start with the breath for stress reduction. But since the ventilator was breathing for him, I could not give cues to slow and deepen the breath for relaxation. Ventilators are set at a certain rate and depth of breath that cannot be changed by the patient. This was the first time I was seeing a patient who could not voluntarily control their breath nor communicate with me verbally. As I stood by the bed, I wondered what to do.

I decided to use guided imagery. I asked him to imagine he was on a peaceful lake floating safely on an oversized air mattress. He was asked to imagine what his senses perceived, such as what he saw and heard. I suggested that he imagine the smell of the water, a light fresh breeze, the feeling of the sun warming him, cool water under him, along with the sounds of lapping water and birdsongs. I then added the sensation of ripples or gentle waves in the lake, lifting and lowering the air mattress as he floated peacefully. I suggested that he synchronize the movement of the waves with the movement of his chest from the ventilator. He was invited to imagine the ventilator as a comforting massage, such as the waves lapping under his floating air mattress, rather than something threatening.

I was amazed at how quickly he calmed down. He seemed to be "riding" the ventilator instead of fighting it. His heart rate decreased, and he stopped trying to pull tubes out. I also introduced the concept of impermanence, the fact that these tubes were temporary, and offered the perspective that the ventilator's sole function was to help him recuperate. I emphasized that the pain would also pass and was not permanent. Some guided meditation for pain relief was incorporated, which he later told me also helped. When I left the room, he seemed to be more in a calm, healing mode rather than an agitated state.

I include this anecdote to demonstrate how powerful yoga therapy can be. In my career as a physician, my usual remedy post-op was to give more medications for pain and agitation. Medications are certainly needed, but this episode showed me how redirecting the energy and attention of the patient to a beneficial healing mode can be immensely helpful too.

Closing Thoughts

My individual journey in the health profession started with a career as an orthopedic physician assistant for five years, followed by a return to medical school in my late twenties. I choose family practice as my specialty because it allowed me to treat a person holistically, including family and social interactions, instead of focusing on one body part or system.

Yoga naturally drew me in when I was introduced to it in my forties. Yoga worked the body, relaxed the mind, and encouraged my spiritual development. My response to the practice of yoga spilled over into my interactions with others. Having my medical background helped me appreciate the anatomical and physiological benefits. The actual practice of yoga helped me appreciate the mental and spiritual benefits, too.

Teaching yoga has allowed me to see that a negative attitude in life can be self-perpetuating and contagious, bringing down those around you. Conversely, a positive attitude can promote health and be even more powerful, allowing people in proximity to feel your energy of enthusiasm, joy, compassion, and contentment. I do not mean to imply that people who practice yoga and meditation are on a constant, even keel of bliss. Positivity, mindfulness, and kindness are intermittent for most of us, but with practice may become more ingrained habitual traits. Humans struggle daily with egos and ignorance, aversions, and desires. Yoga gives humanity tools to cope with these struggles, tools that have been handed down for thousands of years. The practice has survived throughout its long history because it works.

In choosing the title of *Yoga as Integrative Medicine,* I intended two uses of the term "integrative." The first connotation applies to the specialty of integrative medicine, to encourage the use of yoga with traditional Western medical care, along with other modalities, for more holistic care. Scientific studies are starting to document the benefits that countless yogis have taught for generations. I anticipate more research being done on the brain-body connections, including the enteric nervous system of the gut, fascial input, telomeres, and epigenomes, and yoga techniques as therapy. Integrating yoga practice with the advances of modern Western medicine can empower the individual to strive towards optimal self-health.

The second connotation of the word "integrative" in my book title applies to how I explained yogic concepts by integrating them with Western medicine concepts. My physician's mindset was the foundation for incorporating my own yoga knowledge; my understanding of yoga was layered onto my ingrained knowledge of anatomy, physiology, Western medical care, and even my Western way of looking at the world. Therefore, I often used medical terms and concepts in this book to explain some of the teachings of yoga. For example, I correlated the neuroendocrine system (nerve supply and hormones) with the chakras, brain wave patterns with yoga *nidra*, and neuroplasticity with meditation practices. The point was to integrate yogic ideas with Western medicine concepts and give validity to the yoga teachings, especially to those readers with a scientific or medical background. At the same time, my intention was for readers with a strong yoga background to be able to integrate some Western medicine concepts into their knowledge of yoga. I also strove to explain concepts using language that most readers could comprehend. Rather than using terminology that might be intimidating or foreign, I wanted to describe yoga in a way to make it accessible to all.

My goal is for readers to embrace yoga to unite body, mind, and spirit into a healthy, fulfilled, content human being. For many people, the benefits start at the physical level, then expand to the mental and emotional aspects. Spiritual benefits develop with continuing practice, including meditation, mindfulness, and the study of concepts such as the *klesha*s, the koshas, and the eightfold path of the *Yoga Sutras*.

Regardless of religious beliefs, the spiritual exploration of self can lead to joy, personal contentment, and improved interactions with the family and community. Integrating yoga therapy with Western medicine may help ease end-of-life transitions, which can be a challenging time for patients and families. If mortality is contemplated and accepted, death may be less frightening and more peaceful. Cherishing the present, instead of dreading the future, becomes a way of living and allows a certain liberation from worry. You are freer to live in the present, precious moments of now.

The word *namaste* is often spoken at the end of a yoga practice and as a greeting in India. It roughly translates to "the spirit and light in me honors and greets the spirit and light in you." *Namaste* is like saying hello with a smile, a friendly spirit, and a blessing in your heart towards the other person. I certainly appreciate the attention of those of you who have read this far and applaud your interest in learning more about yoga. My heartfelt "namaste" to you.

Some Favorite Quotes

"A writer can do nothing for men more necessary, satisfying, than just simply to reveal to them the infinite possibility of their own souls."

~ Walt Whitman

"It's the action, not the fruit of the action, that's important. You have to do the right thing. It may not be in your power, may not be in your time, that there'll be any fruit. But that doesn't mean you stop doing the right thing. You may never know what results come from your action. But if you do nothing, there will be no result."

~ Mahatma Gandhi

"You've got to make choices that make sense for you because there's always going to be somebody who'll think you should do something different."

~ Michelle Obama

"A man cannot be comfortable without his own approval. There is nothing more satisfying than that sense of being completely 'at home' in your own skin. When you achieve that natural state of 'being,' then you can finally look beyond yourself and fully contribute all your talents to the world."

~ Mark Twain

"Learning is the beginning of wealth. Searching and learning is where the miracle process all begins…This means there are no limits on what you can be, have, or do'"

~ Albert Einstein

"Allow yourself to trust joy and embrace it. You will find you dance with everything."

~ Ralph Waldo Emerson

"The hero's journey always begins with the call. One way or another, a guide must come to say, 'Look, you're in Sleepy Land. Wake. Come on a trip. There is a whole aspect of your consciousness, your being, that's not been touched."

~ Joseph Campbell

"Don't let your brain interfere with your heart"

~ Albert Einstein

"The love that you withhold is the pain that you carry"

~ Ralph Waldo Emerson

"Developing inner values is much like physical exercise. The more we train our abilities, the stronger they become. The difference is that, unlike the body, when it comes to training the mind, there is no limit to how far we can go."

~ The Dalai Lama

"Anger is an acid that can do more harm to the vessel in which it is stored than to anything on which it is poured."

~ Mark Twain

"If you want others to be happy, practice compassion. If you want to be happy, practice compassion."

~ The Dalai Lama

"The religion of the future will be a cosmic religion. It should transcend a personal God and avoid dogmas and theology. Covering both the natural and the spiritual, it should be based on a religious sense arising from the experience of all things, natural and spiritual, as a meaningful unity."

~ Albert Einstein

"First, let us light the torch of our awareness and learn again how to drink tea, eat, wash dishes, walk, sit, drive, and work in awareness."

~ Thich Nhat Hanh

"In rivers, the water that you touch is the last of what has passed and the first of that which comes; so with present time."

~ Leonardo da Vinci

"There are two days in the year that we can not do anything, yesterday and tomorrow"

~ Mahatma Gandhi

"When I run after what I think I want, my days are a furnace of stress and anxiety; if I sit in my own place of patience, what I need flows to me, and without pain. From this I understand that what I want also wants me, is looking for me and attracting me. There is a great secret here for anyone who can grasp it."

~ Rumi

Carefully watch your thoughts, for they become your words. Manage and watch your words, for they become your actions. Consider and judge your actions, for they become your habits. Acknowledge and watch your habits, for they become your values. Understand and embrace your values, for they become your destiny."

~ Mahatma Gandhi

"The knowledge that you have emerged wiser and stronger from setbacks means that you are, ever after, secure in your ability to survive. You will never truly know yourself, or the strength of your relationships, until both have been tested by adversity. Such knowledge is a true gift, for all that it is painfully won, and it has been worth more than any qualification I ever earned."

~ J. K. Rowling

"Gratitude is the wine for the soul. Go on. Get drunk."

~ Rumi

"The beginning of freedom is the realization that you are not 'the thinker.' Knowing this enables you to observe the entity. The moment you start watching the thinker, a higher level of consciousness becomes activated. You then begin to realize that there is a vast realm of intelligence beyond thought, that thought is only a tiny aspect of that intelligence. You also realize that all the things that truly matter

— beauty, love, creativity, joy, inner peace—arise from beyond the mind. You begin to awaken."

~ Eckart Tolle

"A diamond is just a lump of coal that stuck to its job."

~ Leonardo da Vinci

"The common eye sees only the outside of things, and judges by that, but the seeing eye pierces through and reads the heart and the soul, finding there capacities which the outside didn't indicate or promise, and which the other kind of eye couldn't detect."

~ Mark Twain

"The color of the object illuminated partakes of the color of that which illuminates it."

~ Leonardo da Vinci

"It is not impermanence that makes us suffer. What makes us suffer is wanting things to be permanent when they are not."

~ Thich Nhat Hanh

"Take care of your body as if you were going to live forever; Take care of your soul as if you were going to die tomorrow."

~ Saint Augustine

"Our joy, peace, and happiness depend very much on our practice of recognizing and transforming habit energies. There are positive habit energies that we have to cultivate, and negative habit energies that we have to recognize, embrace, and transform. The energy with which we do these things is mindfulness."

~ Thich Nhat Hanh

"Peace and war begin at home. If we truly want peace in the world, let us begin by loving one another in our own families. If we want to spread joy, we need for every family to have joy."

~ Mother Teresa

"Once you have identified with some form of negativity, you do not want to let it go, and on a deeply unconscious level, you do not want positive change. It would threaten your identity as a depressed, angry or hard-done by person. You will then ignore, deny or sabotage the positive in your life. This is a common phenomenon. It is also insane."

~ Eckart Tolle

"We see the world piece by piece, as the sun, the moon, the animal, the tree; but the whole, of which these are the shining parts, is the soul."

~ Ralph Waldo Emerson

Personal mantras

"Instead of no pain, no gain…yoga is about nurture, not torture."

"I pause for butterflies."

"Lead with an open heart."

"Gratitude is the gateway to positive emotions of the heart."

"What you practice becomes stronger."

I am so grateful for all the encouragement given to me by friends and family as I tackled this project. Next time please talk me out of it.

Thanks to all who have been part of my yoga journey – teachers, fellow practitioners, students, employers, friends, class participants, private clients, and referring healthcare providers. You have all formed me into who I am today.

Much thanks and love to my parents for making me possible and a wonderful childhood, and to all my family for memories and so much love. To my children and grandchildren, love will forever link us in our hearts and spirits.

To my husband Ed, thank you for our children and the opportunity to retire early from my medical practice. This beautiful gift of time allowed me to pursue my passion for knowledge and yoga.

Deep gratitude to all my friends and family who contributed feedback, starting with the painfully rough first draft. Your precious time, suggestions, and encouragement helped birth this book. Special thanks to Sheila Honig and Shane Ledford, who read multiple versions of the manuscript, for your invaluable help.

My thanks to Marilyn McSpadden and Kelsey Kraemer for their contributions to this book.

For editorial assistance, my thanks to Angela Nicolosi, Dr. Tim McCall, Connie Ward, and Kelly Birch, for the gradual evolution towards an improved manuscript. Any mistakes or errors, though unintentional, are mine due to misinterpretation or ignorance.

Most of all thanks to the long lineage of yogis who have passed on their knowledge for the benefit of future generations. Let us keep the chakras and nadis glowing on the shoulders of these giants.

Glossary

Abhinivesa - clinging to our way of life, fear of death

Adrenal glands - responsible for secretion of epinephrine, norepinephrine, and cortisol

Afferent nerve – traveling from the body to the spinal cord and brain, sending information

Ahimsa - non-violence

Ajna chakra - called the third eye, located around the forehead or brain, perception, intelligence

Anahata chakra - heart area, positive emotions

Anandamaya kosha - bliss layer surrounding Atman

Annamaya kosha - physical self

Apana vayu - downward movement of energy in the body

Aparigraha - non-grasping

Asana - posture

Asmita – identifying ourselves with the thinking mind or ego

Asteya - non-stealing

Atman - soul

Autonomic Nervous System (ANS) – responsible for the unconscious control and regulation of multiple body functions

Avidya - ignorance

Ayurveda - holistic medical system originating in India

Bandhas - techniques to control the flow of energy in the body

Bhramari – a relaxing breath technique involving humming, bee breath

Bhagavad Gita - story of Arjuna and Krishna with philosophical discussions, part of the *Upanishads*

Brahmacarya - sensual restraint

Celiac Ganglion – part of the celiac plexus, or solar plexus, a complex collection of nerve fibers

Chakras - wheels of energy communicating with pingala, ida, and sushumna

Corpus callosum - area of the brain that connects right and left hemispheres

Dharana - concentration

Dhyana - contemplation

Doshas - Three sets of traits used in ayurvedic medicine: kapha, pitta, and vata

Dvesa - aversion

EEGs - electroencephalograms recording brain wave amplitude and frequency

Efferent Nerves – traveling from the brain and spinal cord to the body, sending commands

Eightfold Path of Yoga - from the *Yoga Sutras*, path to enlightenment, includes the yamas, niyamas, asana, pranayama, pratyahara, dharana, dhyana, and samadhi

Enteric Nervous System - part of the ANS in the gut dealing with the digestion, immune function, and hormone production

Epigenetics – The study of how behavior effects whether genes are turned on or off

Fascia - connective tissue providing support, sensation, and communication throughout the body

Gray's Anatomy - a classic text on anatomy

Gunas - three qualities in nature: tamas, rajas, sattva

Ida – left-sided longitudinal nadi representing lunar, female, coolness, parasympathetic functions

Jalandhara bandha - chin lock to control the flow of energy

kapha - one of the dosha types, represented by earth and water

Kleshas - causes of suffering which include ignorance, ego, aversion, attachment, fear of death

Koshas - components of an individual: physical, energetic, mental, intelligence, and spirit

Ishvara pranidhana - surrender to the universe

Manipura chakra - solar plexus area, drive, ambition

Manomaya kosha – mental self

Mula bandha - engagement of pelvic floor muscles to keep energy from escaping downward

Muladhara chakra - root area, stability, safety, physical needs

Nadis - energetic channels, three primaries are sushumna, pingala, and ida

Niyamas - personal observances

Neuroplasticity - ability of the brain to create new brain cells and neural pathways

Osteoporosis - loss of the bone structure, increasing the potential for fractures

Parasympathetic Nervous System - the rest-and-digest part of the ANS, promotes healing/immunity

Patanjali - author credited with the *Yoga Sutras*

Phrenic nerve - innervates the diaphragm

Pingala – right-sided longitudinal nadi representing solar, male, heating, sympathetic functions

Pitta - one of the dosha types, represented by fire and water

Prana - energy, breath, life-force

Prana vayu - movement of energy governing inhalation and sensory input

Pranamaya kosha - energetic self

Pranayama - the study or control of the breath

Pratyahara – mental withdrawal from distraction of the senses

Rajas - passion, action, drive

Raga - attachment

Sahasrara chakra - crown area, connection with the divine

Samadhi - bliss

Samana vayu - movement of energy inward in the body

Samskaras - ingrained habitual patterns of thought

Sanskrit - a language from India

Santosha - contentment

Sattva - harmony, goodness, positivity

Satya - truthfulness

Saucha - cleanliness

Sitali - a cooling style of breath over a curled tongue

Sushumna - central nadi connecting the chakras, correlates with the spinal cord and brain

Svadhisthana chakra - pelvic area, sensuality, relationships

Svadhyaya - self-study

Sympathetic Nervous System - the fight-or-flight part of the ANS

Tamas - impure, destructive, ignorant

Tapas - effort

Udana vayu - upward movement of energy in the body

Uddiyana bandha - engaging the lower abdominal muscles to direct energy

Ujjayi - style of breath using mildly constricted vocal cords

Upanishads - part of the *Vedic* scriptures, includes the *Bhagavad Gita*

Vata - one of the dosha types, represented by air and space

Vayus - subdivisions of vata, movement and direction of flow of energy in the body

Vishuddha chakra - throat area, confidence, expression, speech

Vyana vayu - movement of energy outward from center of the body

Yamas - social restraints

Yoga Nidra - yoga sleep, a practice of setting intentions and releasing negative thought patterns

Yoga Sutras - a book of aphorisms regarding the teachings of yoga by Patanjali

Upanishads - part of the *Vedas*

Vedas - collection of various Hindu scriptures starting in ancient India

Vijnanamaya kosha - intelligent wisdom self

References

[i] National Center for Complementary and Integrative Health. Complementary, Alternative, or Integrative Health: what's in a name? July 2018 NCCIH Web site. Accessed December 22, 2020

[ii] Keller, Doug. *Heart of the Yogi.* Do Yoga Productions, 2002, p223-230.

[iii] Mccall, Timothy. *Yoga as Medicine the Yoga Prescription for Health and Healing.* Banton Dell, 2007, p28.

[iv] White, David Gordon. *The Yoga Sutra of Patanjali A Biography.* Princeton University Press, 2014, p 18-32.

[v] Goldberg, Phillip. *American Veda.* Harmony Books, 2010, p26-42, p270-271

[vi] White, *The Yoga Sutra of Patanjali.* p109-115.

[viii] Yogi Svatmarama. *Hatha Yoga Pradipika*

[ix] Goldberg. *American Veda.* p 206-209

[x] Sivananda Yoga Vedanta Center. *Practical Ayurveda.* DK, 2018, p 48-49.

[xi] Lad, Vasant. *Textbook of Ayurveda, Vol 1 Fundamental Principles of Ayurveda.* The Ayurvedic Press, 2002, p45-78.

[xii] www.wasatchayurvedaandyoga.com/the-15-subdoshas. Accessed Nov 13, 2021.

[xiv] www.ayurveda-badems.com/the-five-subdoshas-of-pitta. Accessed Nov 13, 2021.

[xv] www.wasatchayurvedaandyoga.com/the-15-subdoshas. Accessed Nov 13, 2021.

[xvii] Hankey, Alex. Ayurvedic Physiology and Etiology: Ayurvedo Amritanaam. The Doshas and Their Functioning in Terms of Contemporary Biology and Physical Chemistry. Journal of alternative and complementary medicine, (New York, N.Y.) Nov 2001, p 567-74.

xviii Minihane, Anne M. et al. Low-grade inflammation, diet composition and health: current research evidence and its translation. Br J Nutr. 2015 Oct 14;114(7):999-1012. doi: 10.1017/S0007114515002093. Epub 2015 Jul 31. PMID: 26228057; PMCID: PMC4579563.

xix Margolis KG, Cryan JF, Mayer EA. The Microbiota-Gut-Brain Axis: From Motility to Mood. Gastroenterology, 2021 Apr;160(5):1486-1501. doi: 10.1053/j.gastro.2020.10.066. Epub 2021 Jan 22. PMID: 33493503.

xx Lokhorst, Gert-Jan, "Descartes and the Pineal Gland". *The Stanford Encyclopedia of Philosophy* (Winter 2021 Edition), Edward N. Zalta (ed.).

xxi Corballis MC. Left brain, right brain: facts and fantasies. PLoS Biol. 2014 Jan;12(1): e1001767. doi: 10.1371/journal.pbio.1001767. Epub 2014 Jan 21. PMID: 24465175; PMCID: PMC3897366.

xxii Haines, Duane e. et el. "human nervous system". Encyclopedia Britannica, 9 Apr. 2020, www.britannica.com/science/human-nervous-system. Accessed 12 November 2021.

xxiii Sharabi AF, Lui F. Anatomy, Abdomen and Pelvis, Splanchnic Nerves. 2021 Aug 11. In: StatPearls [Internet]. Treasure Island (FL): StatPearls Publishing; 2021 Jan–. PMID: 32809339.

xxv Cornman-Homonoff J, Holzwanger DJ, Lee KS, Madoff DC, Li D. Celiac Plexus Block and Neurolysis in the Management of Chronic Upper Abdominal Pain. *Semin Intervent Radiol*, 2017;34(4):376-386. doi:10.1055/s-0037-1608861.

xxvi Benarroch, E.E. Sympathetic System: Overview. in Encyclopedia of the Neurological Sciences (Second Edition), 2014, p 372-375.

xxvii Waxenbaum JA, Reddy V, Varacallo M. Anatomy, Autonomic Nervous System. [Updated 2021 Jul 29]. In: StatPearls [Internet]. Treasure Island (FL): StatPearls Publishing; 2021 Jan-. Available from: www.ncbi.nlm.nih.gov/books/NBK539845.

xxix Oliver KA, Ashurst JV. Anatomy, Thorax, Phrenic Nerves. [Updated 2021 Jul 26]. In: StatPearls [Internet]. Treasure Island (FL): StatPearls Publishing; 2021 Jan-. Available from: www.ncbi.nlm.nih.gov/books/NBK513325.

xxxi Verlinden, T.J.M., van Dijk, P., Herrler, A. *et al.* The human phrenic nerve serves as a morphological conduit for autonomic nerves and innervates the caval body of the diaphragm. *Sci Rep* **8,** 11697 (2018). www.doi.org/10.1038/s41598-018-30145-x.

xxxii www.scottsdaleneurofeedback.com/services/qeeg-brain-mapping/eeg-brainwaves/beta-waves. Accessed Nov 13, 2021.

xxxiii www.healthline.com/health/gamma-brain-waves#bottom-line. Accessed Nov 13, 2021.

xxxiv Lutz A, Greischar LL, Rawlings NB, Ricard M, Davidson RJ. Long-term meditators self-induce high-amplitude gamma synchrony during mental practice. *Proc Natl Acad Sci U S A.* 2004;101(46):16369-16373. doi:10.1073/pnas.0407401101.

xxxv Goleman, Daniel, Davidson, Richard J. *Altered Traits: Science Reveals How Meditation Changes Your Mind, Brain, and Body.* Avery Publishing Group, 2017.

xxxvi Lustenberger C, Boyle MR, Foulser AA, Mellin JM, Fröhlich F. Functional role of frontal alpha oscillations in creativity. Cortex: a Journal Devoted to the Study of the Nervous System and Behavior. 2015 Jun; 67:74-82. DOI: 10.1016/j.cortex.2015.03.012. PMID: 25913062; PMCID: PMC4451406.

xxxvii Theta Brain Waves: 4 Hz To 8 Hz - Mental Health Daily /2014/04/12.

xxxviii www.anahana.com/en/yoga/yoga-nidra. Accessed Nov 13, 2021.

xxxixwww.mentalhealthdaily.com/2014/04/15/5-types-of-brain-waves-frequencies-gamma-beta-alpha-theta-delta. Accessed Nov 13, 2021.

xl Kumar, Kamakhya, Joshi, Bhanu. Study on the effect of Pranakarshan pranayama and Yoga nidra on alpha EEG & GSR. Indian Journal of Traditional Knowledge Vol. 8 (3), July 2009, pp. 453-454.

xli Kjaer T. W., Bertelsen C., Piccini P., Brooks D., Alving J., Lou H. C. Increased dopamine tone during meditation-induced change of consciousness. *Cognitive Brain Research.* 2002;13(2):255–259. doi: 10.1016/S0926-6410(01)00106-9.

xliii Harkess, K., Ryan, J., Delfabbro, P. et al. Preliminary indications of the effect of a brief yoga intervention on markers of inflammation and DNA methylation in chronically stressed women. Transl Psychiatry 6, e965 (2016). https://doi.org/10.1038/tp.2016.234.

xliv Robin, Mel. A Physiological Handbook for Teachers of Yogasana. Fenestra Books, 2002, p 370-373.

xlv Raghuraj P, Telles S. Immediate effect of specific nostril manipulating yoga breathing practices on autonomic and respiratory variables. Appl Psychophysiol Biofeedback. 2008 Jun;33(2):65-75. doi: 10.1007/s10484-008-9055-0. Epub 2008 Mar 18. PMID: 18347974.

xlvi Zaccaro A, Piarulli A, Laurino M, Garbella E, Menicucci D, Neri B, Gemignani A. How Breath-Control Can Change Your Life: A Systematic Review on Psycho-Physiological Correlates of Slow Breathing. Front Hum Neurosci. 2018 Sep 7; 12:353. doi: 10.3389/fnhum.2018.00353. PMID: 30245619; PMCID: PMC6137615.

xlvii Bhavanani AB, Sanjay Z, Madanmohan Immediate effect of sukha pranayama on cardiovascular variables in patients of hypertension. Int J Yoga Therap. 2011; 21:73–6. [PubMed] [Google Scholar].

xlviii Kannan, K, et al. Effectiveness of Pranayama on Depression in Elderly. Journal of Krishna Institute of Medical Sciences Univ. Vol. 4 No. 1, Jan-Mar 2015 Page 18-27.

xlix Sharma VK, M R, S V, Subramanian SK, Bhavanani AB, Madanmohan, Sahai A, Thangavel D. Effect of fast and slow pranayama practice on cognitive functions in healthy volunteers. J Clin Diagn Res. 2014 Jan;8(1):10-3. doi: 10.7860/JCDR/2014/7256.3668. Epub 2013 Nov 18. PMID: 24596711; PMCID: PMC3939514.

l Saoji AA, Raghavendra BR, Manjunath NK. Effects of yogic breath regulation: A narrative review of scientific evidence. J Ayurveda Integr Med. 2019 Jan-Mar;10(1):50-58. doi: 10.1016/j.jaim.2017.07.008. Epub 2018 Feb 1. PMID: 29395894; PMCID: PMC6470305.

li www.nccih.nih.gov/health/meditation-in-depth. Accessed Nov 13, 2021.

lii Bhasin MK, Dusek JA, Chang BH, Joseph MG, Denninger JW, Fricchione GL, Benson H, Libermann TA. Relaxation response induces temporal transcriptome changes in energy metabolism, insulin secretion and inflammatory pathways. PLoS One. 2013 May 1;8(5): e62817. doi: 10.1371/journal.pone.0062817. Erratum in: PLoS One. 2017 Feb 21;12 (2): e0172873. PMID: 23650531; PMCID: PMC3641112.

liii Epel, Blackburn et al, Accelerated telomere shortening in response to life stress, Proc Natl Acad Science USA 2004 Dec 7, 101.

liv Epel, Blackburn et al, Intensive meditation training, immune cell telomerase activity, and psychological mediators, Psychoneuroendocrinology 2011 June 36(5) p 664-81.

lv Schutte & Malouff, "A Mete-Analytic Review of the Effects of Mindfulness Meditation on Telomerase Activity" Psychoneuroendocrinology 42 (2014): p45.

lvi Tonya & Jacobs et al, "Intensive Meditation Training, Immune Cell Telomerase Activity, and Psychological Mediators" Psychoneuroendocrinology 36:5 (2011) 664-81.

lvii Hoge et al, "Loving-Kindness Meditation Practice Associated with Longer Telomeres in Women" Brain, Behavior, and Immunity 32 (2013) 159-63.

lviii Stahl, James E., Dossett, Michelle L., LaJoie, A. Scott, Denninger, John W., Mehta, Darshan H., Goldman, Roberta, Fricchione, Gregory L., Benson, Herbert. Relaxation Response and Resiliency Training and Its Effect on Healthcare Resource Utilization. PLoS One. 2015 October 13; 10.13710.

lix Holzel et al published "Mindfulness practice leads to increases in regional brain gray matter density" (Psychiatry Research Neuroimaging Jan 13th, 2011, Volume 191 pages 36-43).

lx Manna et al. Neural correlates of focused awareness and cognitive monitoring in meditation, Brain Research Bulletin Vol 82 April 29,2010.

lxi Goleman, Davidson, Richard J. *Altered Traits: Science Reveals How Meditation Changes Your Mind, Brain, and Body.* 2017 Penguin Random House p 121, 273-274.

CPSIA information can be obtained
at www.ICGtesting.com
Printed in the USA
LVHW032121121221
706021LV00001B/6